# Bargaining Power

Verna Smith

# Bargaining Power

Health Policymaking from England
and New Zealand

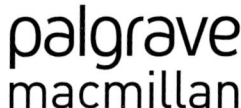

Verna Smith
School of Government
Victoria University of Wellington, School of Government
Wellington, New Zealand

ISBN 978-981-10-7601-5        ISBN 978-981-10-7602-2   (eBook)
https://doi.org/10.1007/978-981-10-7602-2

Library of Congress Control Number: 2017962762

Cover illustration: Pattern adapted from an Indian cotton print produced in the 19th century

Printed on acid-free paper

This Palgrave Pivot imprint is published by Springer Nature
The registered company is Springer Nature Singapore Pte Ltd.
The registered company address is: 152 Beach Road, #21-01/04 Gateway East, Singapore 189721, Singapore

# FOREWORD

To say that policymaking is complex and messy is to state the obvious. Figuring out in what ways and how outcomes are affected by complexity and messiness is far more difficult, especially when one engages in comparative longitudinal research. Dr Smith courageously attempts to do just that. The end product is a solid piece of academic research on the politics of health-care reforms in two national settings: New Zealand and the United Kingdom (more specifically, England as responsibility for the National Health Service has been devolved, to an extent, to Wales and Scotland).

The Multiple Streams Framework (MS Framework) is perhaps the best-known analytical lens to take policy messiness seriously. It centres on five elements: policies, politics, problems, policy windows, policy entrepreneurs. The main argument is that policy choice is more likely when entrepreneurs are able to "sell" their pet policy solutions and problems to interested policymakers operating in the broader polity during open windows of opportunity. The argument is synthetic in that it utilises elements from both structure and agency to provide a complete explanation of policy change. It is also probabilistic in that it speaks in terms of fluctuating chances and increasing likelihoods. But it is also limited in that it leaves out, as the author reminds us, or better yet does not make fully explicit, three key elements of policy: institutional topography, variation in entrepreneurial activity, and policy outcomes (not just outputs). It is important to take them into account but also very difficult to fully and clearly specify their consequences, largely because effects differ over time and across countries.

Better theories of the policy process are far more likely to be built through astute observation and careful empirical verification. Even better are those which attempt to do so comparatively. It is not enough to say institutions matter. One must also specify how, when, and in what national environments. For instance, does centralisation of health care affect the likelihood of raising health-care reform as a salient and important public issue? Does it affect the trajectory of specific alternatives as they make their way through policy networks to soften up? Is it likely to have a greater impact on one or both of these tasks? In one or more countries? If so, how and why?

The same can be said about policy entrepreneurs. Perhaps this is the most difficult element to identify and fully model in any policy framework. We all know that behind great ideas stand great people, meaning that pushing ideas through the maze of government institutions necessitates the presence of well-connected individuals who will argue for the idea, who will make compromises, and who will frame it in ways that appeal to powerful decision-makers. This is difficult not simply because of the level and quality of necessary skills but also because of the time and effort needed. Chances are the idea will not be adopted because important deadlines may be missed, policymakers ignored, or just dumb luck—no one is paying—or wants to pay—attention. Persistence and resources are essential components of success. The MS Framework argues they are important, but who are these entrepreneurs and are they interchangeable? Despite 35 years of research, we still don't know enough. Dr Smith adds one more variant to the already proposed entrepreneurial mix: institutional entrepreneurs. They are individuals who operate within specific institutions—that is, they are not outsiders to the policy at hand—and who take risks to bring about change in a specific direction. Successfully doing so involves balancing two important and difficult tasks relating to process and substance. On the one hand, entrepreneurs must create, maintain, and enhance support for the idea (policy) in both the political and public spheres. On the other hand, they must be careful to compromise, but not too much, so as to retain the basic policy design that addresses a given problem. The two tasks are autonomous but linked in the sense they involve different dynamics which also affect one another. In this way, entrepreneurial activity is not just a risk-taking exercise in terms of policy but also a balancing exercise in terms of the various risks involved.

Finally, a major limitation is MS Framework's inattention to policy outcomes. It is not enough to examine how issues rise and fall on the government's agenda. It is not enough to explain why one policy was adopted among many others. We must also look at how specific policies affect the social conditions they are designed to affect in order to understand the full public policy cycle. Social effects often become the requisite demands later for more (or less) policy change. They contribute to our understanding of why some issues remain on the government agenda for a very long time while others fade away rather quickly.

Fully specifying these dynamics is a Herculean task in any national environment. Trying to do this comparatively is even more difficult because it necessitates a clever research design to keep some variables constant while allowing the factors of interest to vary. Because most social science, and certainly this study, operates in quasi-experimental conditions where control of the environment is very limited, policy analysis is complex and messy regardless of analytical lens. Dr Smith has taken on this challenge with care and enthusiasm. I invite the reader to pass judgement whether this was done successfully, but more importantly to replicate, debate and, if necessary, amend the findings. For the true hallmark of good academic work is not for the author to demonstrate he/she is right—that is by definition the point of doing research. Good research invites replication and confirmation (or not) of the findings. The author has done her job provocatively well. Will others take on this challenge?

Rhodes College                                              Nikolaos Zahariadis
Memphis, TN, USA

# PREFACE AND ACKNOWLEDGEMENTS

I have long believed that a strong state and a strong medical profession working together could deliver policies which reduce health disparities and improve health outcomes for citizens. I was therefore keen to study two pay-for-performance schemes introduced in the primary health-care systems of England and New Zealand between 2001 and 2007, hoping that, through comparative study, I could draw out lessons for today's policymakers. Starting my research in 2007, I also wanted to test whether the multi-theoretic Multiple Streams Framework of John Kingdon, as it has been interpreted and adapted by Zahariadis (2007), explained what happened in these two policymaking episodes better than single-theory explanations for policy change and variation.

In setting this book in two countries I have drawn upon a long and deep sense of connection to England as well as to the country of my birth, New Zealand. My research reflects this fascination with both countries and the similarities and differences in their responses to one of the great policymaking challenges of our times: to achieve improved health outcomes for their citizens. In writing this book, I have been delighted and humbled by the generous support which I have received from the policymakers of both countries involved in this research, whether they were general practitioners or primary health-care professionals, civil servants, senior politicians or health researchers, and I thank them most sincerely for this. I owe special thanks to Professor Jacqueline Cumming of Victoria University of Wellington and Professor Judith Smith of the University of Birmingham for guiding this research with rigour and great care. Professor Michael Mintrom of Monash University has also provided invaluable advice, support and encouragement. I thank them all deeply for delivering this over many years. I also thank Janet Keilar and Vic Lipski for their invaluable help with preparing this book for publication.

Finally, the encouragement of my friends in England and New Zealand, their support of my decision to begin the research, their constant interest in progress, and their acceptance that my social life had to be dramatically curtailed for years while I completed this research kept me going. This book is dedicated to them.

Wellington, New Zealand                                           Verna Smith

## REFERENCE

Zahariadis, N. (2007). The Multiple Streams Framework. In P. A. Sabatier (Ed.), *Theories of the Policy Process*. Boulder: Westview Press.

# CONTENTS

1 A Tale of Two Countries                                                    1

2 Analysing Public Policy: Does Kingdon's Multiple
  Streams Framework Help?                                                    9

3 A Comparison of the English and New Zealand
  General Practice Sub-Systems                                              21

4 England: Context and the Quality and Outcomes
  Framework                                                                 33

5 Utility of Kingdon's Framework: Policymaking
  in England                                                                59

6 New Zealand: Context and the Performance
  Programme                                                                 75

7 Utility of Kingdon's Framework: Policymaking
  in New Zealand                                                           111

8    The Two Case Studies Compared                    125

9    Conclusion                                       153

Appendix                                             157

References                                           161

Index                                                171

# Acronyms

| | |
|---|---|
| BMA | British Medical Association |
| DHB | District Health Board |
| GP | General practice/general practitioner |
| GPC | General Practitioners Committee |
| IPA | Independent Practitioners' Association |
| MPIG | Minimum Practice Income Guarantee |
| MS | Multiple Streams [Framework] |
| NHS | National Health Service |
| No. 10 | Prime Minister's Office and Residence, London |
| NZLP | New Zealand Labour Party |
| NZMA | New Zealand Medical Association |
| PCT | Primary Care Trust |
| PHCS | Primary Health-Care Strategy |
| PHO | Primary Health Organisation |
| PHONZ | Primary Health Organisations New Zealand |
| PP | Performance Programme |
| PRICCE | Primary Care Clinical Effectiveness |
| QMAS | Quality Management Advisory System |
| QOF | Quality and Outcomes Framework |
| RSAG | Referred Services Advisory Group |
| RSEAG | Referred Services Expert Advisory Group |

# LIST OF TABLES

Table 3.1   General practice systems: England and New Zealand—key
            features and changes during reform period                    28
Table 8.1   The two case studies compared: drivers analysis for
            pay-for-performance policymaking                             126

CHAPTER 1

# A Tale of Two Countries

**Abstract** Policymakers need to know why policy changes or varies between sectors or countries, to improve their ability to design effective policies. This compelling comparative analysis of two case studies of pay-for-performance policymaking within general practice in similar countries, England and New Zealand, uncovers the drivers of each policymaking process and the reasons for differing outcomes. An innovative analytical framework is introduced, testing the comparative utility of single-approach theories that cite the influence of institutions, interest groups, the rational choices made by individuals, ideas or socio-economic factors, and a multi-theoretic approach, John Kingdon's Multiple Streams Framework.

**Keywords** Policy change and variation • Multiple Streams Framework • Pay-for-performance

In the years following 2000, the governments of England[1] and New Zealand each made major changes to the governance and financing arrangements for their general practice services. The reforms were designed, among other things, to give state funders greater influence over the medical profession's responsibility for quality and allocation of publicly funded health care, increasing the clinical and financial accountability of general practitioners to the state (King 2001 p. 11; Stevens 2004). Each country introduced a pay-for-performance scheme for general practitioners. The design of these schemes differed in size, scope and speed of implementation; consequently, the two schemes are associated with differing levels of impact upon health outcomes.

Policymakers need to know why and how policy change occurs, and why the processes or outcomes of policymaking differ between countries, in order to improve their ability to bring policy change. In the public policy literature, scholars debate whether the influence of institutions, interest groups, individuals' rational choices, ideas or socio-economic factors are the main drivers of policy change and variation. Does structure or agency dominate in this process? Is it institutions or people who need to change in order for policy to change? John sets out five approaches or theories that can explain how policy is made and implemented (John 1998). First, institutionalist approaches emphasise the determining role of political organisations and the rules, norms and strategies associated with them. Group-based approaches contend that change arises through the interaction of institutional arrangements and groups or networks, through collective action. Rational choice explanations for policy change focus on the preferences and rational choices of individual actors. Ideas and their advocacy by actors are thought to be the primary driver of policy change by ideational theorists, transcending the influence of political institutions and interests. Finally, socio-economic theories suggest that objective social and economic conditions structure policy formation and therefore drive policy change. John finds that these single-theory approaches fail to explain policy change and variation adequately and contends that multi-theoretic approaches, such as John Kingdon's Multiple Streams Framework (hereafter the MS Framework) (Kingdon 2010), with its mix of explanatory drivers, have greater utility to explain complex policymaking (John 1998, p. 167).

This book presents a new analytical approach. The approach synthesises all five single-theory explanations of policy change and the MS Framework into a coherent approach to assessing policy change and variation. It tests this approach through comparative analysis of policy change and variation in two similar pay-for-performance policymaking case studies in two similar structural and well-established institutional settings. The MS Framework is widely used by scholars (Jones 2015); the research underlying this book, completed in 2014, seeks to make a significant contribution to its refinement by using the insights from this research to test the respective utility of all five elements of the Framework and the sub-elements identified by

Zahariadis (2007), along with the five other single-theory explanations for policy change and variation, to explain the policy change and variation which occurred. It makes recommendations for adaptation of the MS Framework on the basis of these findings.

## THE SETTING

It can be said that "experimental" conditions existed between 2001 and 2007 in England and New Zealand, enabling the comparative study of these contemporaneous, similar policymaking episodes. The countries share similar political and health systems, an earlier similar pattern of health system establishment and a recent history of its reform, involving the application of New Public Management approaches. Both have similar majoritarian, unitary political systems with adversarial features (in which at least two parties oppose each other vigorously on matters relating to the state and the general welfare of the people; Pollitt 2010). In these systems the central government is ultimately supreme, unlike federal states (such as the USA) in which sub-national units such as states share sovereignty with the central government and have powers that the central government may not unilaterally alter. Britain has a majoritarian parliament, typically giving a majority of seats to the party with a plurality of votes in constituencies (a "first past the post" system). New Zealand had the same electoral system until 1996, when a version of proportional representation was introduced. The high executive autonomy (Mulgan 1995; Richards 2002; Shaw 2008) in both countries generally delivers strong majority government that empowers a Cabinet to make policy, often without constraint by the legislature (Blank 2006).

The national health systems of the countries are similar and are often listed in the same categories of health system typologies (OECD 1987; Laugesen 2000; Scott 2001; Burau 2006; Gauld 2009; Tenbensel 2011), having taxpayer-funded national health services in which comprehensive health services are available to all citizens. Established between 1938 and 1948, they are largely publicly funded: in 2000, 80.9 per cent of health expenditure in Britain was public and 78 per cent in New Zealand (OECD 2004, p. 268). Funding is pooled, centrally managed and allocated prospectively in annual budget appropriations. In this respect they are both national health systems in the OECD 1987 typology (OECD 1987).

Docteur and Oxley (OECD 2004, p. 22) note that the extent of public versus private coverage affects the degree of government control over health spending. Whereas the English general practice sub-system has strong hierarchical features, enabling periodic abrupt and dramatic change ordered from the top (Tuohy 1999, p. 14), New Zealand has a complex mix of ownership and governance arrangements in the general practice sub-system as a result of its largely privately provided general practice services and is assessed as providing minimal opportunities for public influence (Tuohy 1999; Davis 2000; Gauld 2003; Crampton 2004; Starke 2010; Tuohy 2012).

These differences in financing and provision arrangements and mechanisms for accountability in the general practice sub-systems create different problems for each overarching health system. The need for more preventive and population-based primary health care, better provision in isolated areas and less variation in quality of treatment is common to both countries. However, England also has concerns about access to services, quality and levels of responsiveness to patient needs and expectations, particularly waiting times for treatment. In New Zealand, high patient charges are the major concern, deterring needed visits to the doctor (Cumming 2002, 2011). New Zealand policymakers have few levers to encourage general practitioners to keep costs of consultations affordable. Each country has taken different approaches to resolve these needs and to improve quality of services. Whereas England developed strong centralised initiatives through its hierarchical system of management of the national health service and close working relationship between the state and the profession, in New Zealand a "stand-off between government and general practitioners" (Crampton 2000, p. 216) has developed and fewer quality initiatives, emanating largely from peer-led initiatives generated from within the profession, are seen (Seddon 2001).

### History of Approaches to Health Policy Problems

To change the structural and institutional arrangements of a health system requires an effort of significant political will, usually emanating from outside the health arena in rare windows of opportunity (Tuohy 1999, p. 11). Both countries have achieved this several times, from the establishment of their national health systems to a period of reform in the 1990s when both systems were restructured to introduce competitive approaches to enhance efficiency and effectiveness, driven by New Public Management and economic theory (Davis 2000; Pollitt 2011), and again at the turn of this century. Each country's governments have used their substantial financing role to undertake system-wide strategic public policy interventions, assisted by their monopsony powers (Scott 2001, p. 152). Implementation of changes did not always follow smoothly, with aspects of the reforms unravelling in each country (Tuohy 1999; Finlayson 2000).

The parallel nature of the reform pathway between these countries is often noted in the literature (OECD 1994; Tuohy 1999; Mays 2000; Scott 2001; Gauld 2009; Pollitt 2011). They are characterised as "New Public Management-intensive jurisdictions" (Pollitt 2011), having introduced more competition, market-type models and business-like methods within their public sectors and giving a large role for private sector forms and techniques such as quasi-markets, large-scale contracting out, market testing, contractual appointments and performance pay for civil servants (2011, p. 116).

### The Policy Instrument: Pay-for-Performance

Pay-for-performance is the delivery of "financial incentives that reward providers for achievement of a range of payer objectives, including delivery efficiencies, submission of data and measures to [monitor] and improve quality and patient safety" (McNamara 2006; Nolte 2008, p. 3). The literature warns of many barriers to successful implementation of financial incentive schemes with general practitioners, not least of which is the opposition of the medical profession. Other barriers include design issues such as setting bonuses or incentives too small or funding incentives from within existing budgets, applying incentives to too small an area of the general practitioner's work, paying for activities rather than results, paying for standards of quality which are already being met rather than for improvements, replacing the intrinsic motive to do a good job for patients with a financial one and reducing the effort in those areas not incentivized. Financial incentive schemes are regarded as having a high risk that they will be gamed or the benefits will be claimed unfairly. Implementation issues include the availability of adequate data on performance, incurring much more cost than predicted, difficulties in monitoring whether quality improvements have actually occurred and questions over timing of payments, treatment of setup costs for practices and publication of results (Chaix-Coutourier 2000; Epstein 2004; Rosenthal 2005).

The literature on pay-for-performance in primary health care has burgeoned, with 20 systematic reviews and one systematic review of systematic reviews about whether pay-for-performance improves the quality of health care (Roland 2014). The authors of this last work conclude that there is clear evidence that pay-for-performance can be effective but the effects can be short term and often not as large as payers wish, depend on the context and can have unintended consequences. They conclude that it is not whether pay-for-performance should be a component of physician pay, but rather which type of pay-for-performance should be used, and in combination with which other quality improvement interventions.

## NOTES

1. This is a comparison of policymaking in England, rather than the United Kingdom, as some differences in policymaking in health exist between the countries of the United Kingdom subsequent to devolution of political responsibility for the NHS to Scotland and Wales in 1998. However, where research refers to the four countries of the United Kingdom in the thesis, United Kingdom or Britain will be used.

## REFERENCES

Blank, R., & Burau, V. (2006). Setting Health Priorities Across Nations: More Convergence Than Divergence? *Journal of Public Health Policy, 27*(3), 265–281.

Burau, V., & Blank, R. (2006). Comparing Health Policy: An Assessment of Typologies of Health Systems. *Journal of Comparative Policy Analysis, 8*(1), 63–76.

Chaix-Coutourier, C., Durand-Zaleski, I., Jolly, D., & Durieux, P. (2000). Effects of Financial Incentives on Medical Practice: Results from a Systematic Review of the Literature and Methodological Issues. *International Journal for Quality in Health Care, 12*(2), 133–142.

Crampton, P. (2000). Policies for General Practice. In P. Davis & T. Ashton (Eds.), *Health and Public Policy in New Zealand*. Auckland: Oxford University Press.

Crampton, P., Davis, P., Lay-Yee, R., Raymont, A., Forrest, C., & Starfield, B. (2004). Comparison of Private For-profit with Private Community-Governed Not-for-profit Primary Care Services in New Zealand. *Journal of Health Services Research & Policy, 9*(Suppl 2), 17–22.

Cumming, J., & Mays, N. (2002). Reform and Counter Reform: How Sustainable Is New Zealand's Latest Health System Restructuring? *Journal of Health Services Research & Policy, 7*(Suppl 1), 46–55.

Cumming, J., & Mays, N. (2011). New Zealand's Primary Health Care Strategy: Early Effects of the New Financing and Payment System for General Practice and Future Challenges. *Health Economics, Policy and Law, 6*, 1–21.

Davis, P., & Ashton, T. (2000). *Health Policy and Public Policy in New Zealand.* Auckland: Oxford University Press.

Epstein, A., Thomas, H. L., & Hamel, M. B. (2004). Paying Physicians for High Quality Health Care. *New England Journal of Medicine, 350*(4), 406–409.

Finlayson, M. (2000). Policy Implementation and Modification. In P. Davis & T. Ashton (Eds.), *Health and Public Policy in New Zealand.* Auckland: Oxford University Press.

Gauld, R. (2003). One Country, Four Systems: Comparing Changing Helath Policies in New Zealand. *International Political Science Review, 24*(2), 199–218.

Gauld, R. (2009). *The New Health Policy.* Maidenhead: Open University Press.

John, P. (1998). *Analysing Public Policy.* London: Cassell.

Jones, M., Peterson, H., Pierce, J., Herweg, N., Bernal, A., Raney, H. L., et al. (2015). A River Runs Through It: A Multiple Streams Meta-review. *Policy Studies Journal, 44*(1), 13–36.

King, A. (2001). *The Primary Health Care Strategy.* Wellington: Ministry of Health.

Kingdon, J. W. (2010). *Agendas, Alternatives, and Public Policies, Update Edition, with an Epilogue on Health Care.* London: Longmans.

Laugesen, M. (2000). The Institutional Context. In P. Davis & T. Ashton (Eds.), *Health and Public Policy in New Zealand.* Auckland: Oxford University Press.

Mays, N., & Hand, K. (2000). *A Review of Options for Health and Disability Support Purchasing in New Zealand.* Wellington: The Treasury.

McNamara, P. (2006). Foreword: Payment Matters? The Next Chapter. *Medical Care Research Review, 63*(Suppl 1), 5S–10S.

Mulgan, R. (1995). Democratic Failure of a Single Party Government. *Australasian Political Studies Association, 30*, 82–97.

Nolte, E., & McKee, M. (2008). *Caring for People with Chronic Conditions.* Maidenhead: Open University Press.

OECD. (1987). *Financing and Delivering Health Care: A Comparative Analysis of OECD Countries.* Paris: OECD.

OECD. (1994). *The Reform of Health Care Systems.* Paris: OECD.

OECD. (2004). *Towards High Performing Health Systems.* Paris: OECD.

Pollitt, C., & Bouckaert, G. (2011). *Public Management Reform.* Oxford: Oxford University Press.

Pollitt, C., Harrison, S., Dowswell, G., Jerak-Zuiderent, S., & Bal, R. (2010). Performance Regimes in Health Care: Institutions, Critical Junctures and the Logic of Escalation in England and the Netherlands. *Evaluation, 16*(1), 13–29.

Richards, D., & Smith, M. (2002). *Governance and Public Policy in the UK.* Oxford: Oxford University Press.

Roland, M., & Campbell, S. (2014). Successes and Failures of Pay for Performance in the United Kingdom. *New England Journal of Medicine, 370*(20), 1944–1949.

Rosenthal, M., Frank, R. G., Zhongie, L., & Epstein, A. M. (2005). Early Experience with Pay-for-performance. *JAMA, 294*(14), 1788–1793.

Scott, C. (2001). *Public and Private Roles in Health Care Systems*. Buckingham: Open University Press.

Seddon, M. E., Marshall, M. N., Campbell, S. M., & Roland, M. O. (2001). Systematic Review of Studies of Quality of Clinical Care in General Practice in the UK, Australia and New Zealand. *Quality and Safety in Health Care, 10*, 152–158.

Shaw, R., & Eichbaum, C. (2008). *Public Policy in New Zealand*. Auckland: Pearson Education.

Starke, P. (2010). Why Institutions Are Not the Only Thing That Matters: Twenty-Five Years of Health Care Reform in New Zealand. *Journal of Health Politics, Policy and Law, 35*(4), 487–516.

Stevens, S. (2004). Reform Strategies for the English NHS. *Health Affairs, 23*(3), 37–44.

Tenbensel, T., Mays, N., & Cumming, J. (2011). A Successful Mix of Hierarchy and Collaboration? Interpreting the 2001 Reform of the Governance of the New Zealand Public Health System. *Policy & Politics, 39*(2), 239–255.

Tuohy, C. H. (1999). *Accidental Logics*. Oxford: Oxford University Press.

Tuohy, C. H. (2012). *Institutional Entrepreneurs and the Politics of Redesigning the Welfare State: The Case of Health Care*. New Orleans, a paper to be presented at the annual meeting of the American Political Science Association, New Orleans, Louisiana.

Zahariadis, N. (2007). The Multiple Streams Framework. In P. A. Sabatier (Ed.), *Theories of the Policy Process*. Boulder: Westview Press.

# CHAPTER 2

# Analysing Public Policy: Does Kingdon's Multiple Streams Framework Help?

**Abstract** Kingdon's Multiple Streams Framework is a popular multi-theoretic approach which explains non-incremental policy change by synthesising elements from structural and agency-based theories. However, the Framework has attracted much critical commentary, particularly for its neglect of institutional dynamics and the importance of history in policy-making processes. Its five central elements of policies, politics, problems, policy windows and policy entrepreneurs are presented, subsequent enhancements described and examples given of its growing use internationally to explain public policymaking. This research takes on the challenge to test two core hypotheses of the Framework: the conditions required for non-incremental change and the need for policy entrepreneurs to couple three streams at the agenda-setting phase. The findings of the research challenge these hypotheses and make the case for refinement of the Framework.

**Keywords** Multiple Streams Framework • Institutional entrepreneurs • Institutional context • Parliamentary democracies

Public policy research studies "how the machinery of the state and political actors interact to produce public actions" (John 1998, p. 2) in order to understand and improve public policymaking. Because of the complexity of public policymaking, John concludes that multi-theoretic approaches

© The Author(s) 2018
V. Smith, *Bargaining Power*,
https://doi.org/10.1007/978-981-10-7602-2_2

which can explain both constraining forces (such as institutions and patterns of interest group relationships) and driving forces (such as ideas and individual actors) have greater explanatory power for public policy-making than single-theory approaches. John sees the interplay between ideas and interests among actors as the driving force for policy change, structured by the constraining forces of institutions, patterns of interest group or network relationships and socio-economic structures.

One multi-theoretic approach, Kingdon's MS Framework, is regarded by John as the closest to "an adequate theory of public policy." Kingdon's *Agendas, Alternatives and Public Policies* (1984) focused on the processes in public policy agenda-setting that he observed in the USA (Kingdon 2010, pp. 1–3). He challenged the prevailing view that planned, top-down policymaking processes could achieve non-incremental change by providing strong evidence of discontinuity and non-incrementalism, especially in the agenda-setting phase. His theory accommodates the notion that at the alternative generation stage, familiar ideas and approaches may be drawn upon but he considers that agenda-setting is more likely to depend upon chance and the receptivity of the climate (which entrepreneurial actors can manipulate) than on existing policy settings. His MS Framework describes how non-incremental change needs conditions of ambiguity, some element of political manipulation and no clear technology for change. He hypothesised that ideas, actors, institutions, socio-economic circumstances and political interests all interact in this process. The most important features he found were the elements of chance and creativity as hypothesised in the Garbage Can Model of Organisational Choice (Cohen 1972).

## Ambiguity, Fluid Participation and Unclear Technology

The three characteristics of Cohen's Garbage Can Model at the core of Kingdon's theory (Kingdon 2010, p. 84) are problematic (or ambiguous) preferences, fluid participation involving many actors and unclear technology for solving the problem. The first two are often exacerbated by temporal constraints and together these circumstances militate against rational, measured, incremental policymaking. Kingdon observed dramatic non-incremental policy change facilitated by opportunistic policy actors he called "policy entrepreneurs," who were looking for a window of opportunity or "policy window."

Kingdon's famous metaphor of the "policy primeval soup" describes the agenda-setting stage where policy ideas and proposals developed by specialists in a policy community float for selection, are tested for technical feasibility, fit with dominant values and the current national mood, budgetary workability and potential political support or opposition. He describes three live streams flowing independently of one another: policy problems, policy solutions and political processes, such as election results or changes in public opinion. A process of "coupling," often achieved by policy entrepreneurs, is defined by Kingdon as critical. The Framework sets out the relative importance of various actors at different stages of the policymaking process: agenda-setting, alternative selection, decision-making and implementation.

Kingdon finds the president and elected officials (and their appointed officials) to be of greatest importance in agenda-setting. Civil servants and interest groups, including provider groups such as medical professionals, are more important in the alternative selection stage or development of the legislation that is emerging (Kingdon 2010, p. 50). In this phase, policymaking is more likely to be characterised by incremental processes. Interest groups are considered to be more likely to constrain or adapt rather than promote policy ideas. Political influence and internal cohesion are resources held by the policy community which are important to the process. These can, if mobilised, have considerable electoral effect. Academics, researchers, media actors, electoral actors (such as campaigners and political parties) and the opinions of the general public are all important and their influence weighed and explained in Kingdon's model at each of the four stages. Kingdon briefly mentions decision-making and implementation, citing the civil servant actors as critical to the implementation phase and acknowledging that these stages constitute a process which can generate feedback leading to innovation and further policy change. He cites the longevity and technical expertise of civil servants and their well-developed relationships with other key players, particularly those in interest groups, as being key resources of relevance to this phase of the process (Kingdon 2010, p. 31).

Zahariadis (2007; Sabatier 2014) has facilitated empirical analysis of policymaking using the theory by drawing out the five key structural elements in the MS Framework which lead to a policy output. He identifies key features or inputs as sub-elements, which are listed here and explained further below:

| | |
|---|---|
| Problems Stream: | "Indicators," "Focusing Events," "Feedback" and "Load" |
| Politics Stream: | "Party Ideology," "National Mood" and "Balance of Interests" |
| Policy Stream: | "Value acceptability," "Technical Feasibility," "Resource Adequacy" and "Network Integration" |
| Policy Window: | "Coupling Logic," "Decision Style" and "Institutional Context" |
| Policy Entrepreneurs: | "Access," "Resources" and "Strategies" |

## PROBLEMS STREAM

Problems, according to Kingdon, are "conditions that policymakers and citizens want addressed" such as rising medical costs, and they are discovered through "indicators" which may be being monitored routinely or through special studies. Depending on perception and interpretation of any change in that condition shown by the indicator and the beliefs and values associated with it, a condition may come to be seen as a problem. A "focusing event," such as a dramatic failure in quality, may trigger a condition becoming a problem, especially if exacerbated by media attention or the work of policy entrepreneurs. "Feedback" from programmes is another major source of policymakers finding out about conditions. It could be good, which may lead to a programme being replicated ("spill-over") or poor, which may trigger a new policymaking process to change the programme. The "load," or number of difficult problems faced by an administration, will influence whether a condition gets onto a policy agenda.

## POLITICS STREAM

"National mood," "balance of interests" or pressure-group campaigns and attitudes of interest groups to policies, and administrative or legislative turnover are the key elements affecting the Politics Stream according to Zahariadis. Government's soundings of public opinion or concerns expressed by interest groups may promote or dim the issue. Political change such as a change of government provides considerable potential for dealing with problems because the new administration may have different ideas from the previous one and be keen to implement them. "Party Ideology," such as items in electoral manifestos, affects how they will deal with each problem.

## POLICY STREAM

Kingdon described a "soup" of ideas competing to win acceptance in policy communities of bureaucrats, academics and researchers. Zahariadis has deconstructed this high-level description by differentiating between two major subjects for analysis, the policy itself and the policy community around it, which he renames the "network."[1] Each can be analysed according to aspects of "technical feasibility," "resource adequacy" and "value acceptability," and the network can be analysed further according to its level of integration. Only a few ideas are selected for the agenda, which are influenced by their technical feasibility (how easy they are to implement), their congruence with values of policymakers and their cost. However, the type of network of specialists and specifically its level of "integration" (or linkages among participants) is also important to the chances of success in getting items onto the agenda and selected from competing alternatives. This is influenced by the "size" of the network, the nature of participants' "mode" of political exchange, the network's degree of "administrative capacity" and the nature of "access" to key decision-makers within the network or to those seeking membership of the network from outside it. Briefly, he suggests (Zahariadis 1995, pp. 73–75) that networks sit on a continuum from smaller, more integrated ones, having a consensual mode, higher capacity and more restricted access to membership, to larger, less integrated ones, having a competitive mode, lower administrative capacity and less restricted access. Issues and ideas have different trajectories for rising to the top of the soup for selection. Zahariadis suggests that more integrated networks will tend to follow an "emergent to convergent" pattern in which longer periods of consensus-based debate occurs, followed by rapid acceptance and uptake of policy ideas. Less integrated networks will tend to follow a pattern of sudden break-through of ideas, perhaps without attracting much support, followed by gradual steps which soften resistance and move the policy idea towards more broad-based acceptance.

## POLICY WINDOWS

Policy windows present "coupling" opportunities arising as a consequence of a "compelling event" such as a natural disaster or the institutional context, such as election of a new administration with a "doctrinal" reason to make a change in policy. The type of window defines the context in which the policy is made. Where windows open in the Politics Stream such as at administrative turnover, the process is ideological and policies are made in search of a rationale. Policy made in brief windows may create an ongoing path-dependent process of later policymaking. The coupling of problems and solutions depends on the "decision-making style" of the administration in power at the time, with more cautious styles requiring more information.

## Policy Entrepreneurs

In the MS Framework, policy entrepreneurs are key actors or organisations who utilise techniques of political manipulation to gain traction for a policy idea in conditions of ambiguity, enabling non-incremental change. The logic of political manipulation sets this lens apart from others which employ rationality (such as rational choice) or persuasion (Zahariadis 2007, p. 69). Driven perhaps by self-interest, a policy entrepreneur's chance of success is affected by the level of "access" to policymakers, the "resources" (time, money and energy) they have and their skill at using manipulative "strategies," such as "framing" (or putting the case for the policy with a set of meanings suitable to a particular audience) and "salami tactics" (or feeding out the policy ideas bit by bit) to couple the three streams.

## Improving the MS Framework

The MS Framework has been criticised for a number of reasons, including the lack of a testable hypothesis, inability to test it quantitatively, absence of a micro-foundation (or set of assumptions) and, of most relevance for this research, the absence of institutions as an element in the Framework (Zohlnhöfer 2016a, p. 8).

Zahariadis acknowledges that Kingdon has underplayed both institutional dynamics and the importance of history in the MS Framework, and has refined it by incorporating some of these concepts more explicitly in the sub-elements. For instance, "Party Ideology" describes how dramatic policy change can occur in the Politics Stream when administrations change. Zahariadis has also improved the Framework by explaining how the structure and characteristics of policy networks (which are called policy communities in Kingdon's Framework) influence the trajectory of ideas in the Policy Stream (Zahariadis 1995, p. 91) and how long time periods may be relevant. He draws on policy network theory (Marsh 1992) to describe how the mode of exchange or pattern of interaction between participants in the policy network may be quite asymmetrical but "forces interdependent participants to exchange one resource for another without the ability of any one member to single-handedly impose his or her will on the rest" (Zahariadis 1995, p. 75). Consensus-based network modes have a higher degree of integration and contacts are more frequent and more formalised, characterised by bargaining or "sounding out" and compromise. Competitive modes have more infrequent and chaotic contacts between participants and adversarial relationships are more likely. In competitive modes, zero-sum approaches are taken in which the consent of most but not necessarily all participants is gained but subsequent opposition may slow or undermine the policy ideas thus implemented.

Zahariadis (1995, p. 92) also contends the "range of solutions likely to receive a hearing is bounded by history and biased by network structures" (Zahariadis 1995, p. 92). In more integrated networks there is "rapid propulsion to salience of a persistently softened idea" (Zahariadis 1995, p. 73), whereas a less integrated network will display initial "quantum" changes which evolve into a more gradualist pathway. Network size is a factor. Where there are few restrictions to entry, a large and varied membership can develop. Competitive modes of discourse typically dominate large networks and will result in many contending ideas and more adversarial relationships. By contrast, in a more integrated and usually smaller network with restrictions on access to membership but good access to decision-makers, common interests and a search for unanimity among the players place a premium on consensus building, intense bargaining and accommodating amendments to policy. Ideas slowly evolve through these processes until they can rapidly be implemented with widespread support.

The variables of value acceptability and technical feasibility apply to the policy as well as to the policy community. While the policy may in theory be technically feasible it may not actually be feasible to implement in the policy community because of the structure or capacity of the community or a lack of suitable administrative tools. Such tools could be requisite contractual or financing arrangements or appropriate information management infrastructure.

These enhancements of the MS Framework are reflected in the addition by Zahariadis of the sub-elements of "Balance of Interests" to the Politics Stream, "Institutional Context" to the Policy Window and "Network Integration" and "Policy Community" to the Policy Stream in an updated Diagram of the Multiple Streams Framework (Sabatier 2014, p. 36; Jones 2015).

The enhancements made by Zahariadis are most valuable. However, the Framework still pays too little attention to structural and institutional arrangements. The limited emphasis on structural characteristics and decision-making processes of political institutions, which are largely resilient to the turnover of individuals, as a major driver of policy action or inaction, renders the Framework less useful in jurisdictions where these factors are important. Zahariadis contends that "institutions make things possible, but people make things happen" and suggests that this emphasis needs to be rediscovered and explored (Sabatier 2014, p. 45).

Pressure to continue to evolve Kingdon's MS Framework has grown with its popularity as a widely recognised approach to public policymaking used by scholars throughout the world (Jones 2015). It has been applied to 22 different policy arenas and 65 countries, including 53 studies in the United Kingdom and one in New Zealand. The New Zealand study (Aberbach 2001, p. 419) finds similar drivers of non-incremental policy change to those which will be identified in this book. Twenty-eight per cent of the studies considered health policy. It has been applied to health policy change addressing health inequalities in a small case study in Norway and demonstrates the importance of a policy window occurring at a change of government which enables a non-linear shift (Strand 2011). Kusi-Ampofo applies the MS Framework to a Type 1 case study of non-incremental health policymaking in Ghana, studying a change in funding arrangements which was also triggered by a change of government, using a policy evolution analysis method (Kusi-Ampofo 2015).

Much early research inspired by the MS Framework focused on the policy entrepreneur role. Further analysis has identified four central elements shared by all policy entrepreneurs to some extent, namely social acuity, ability to define problems, building teams and leading by example (Mintrom 1996). Mintrom considers that deep knowledge of relevant procedures and local norms within institutions (which he calls "insider sensibilities") can significantly increase the ability of actors to instigate change (Mintrom 2009). Oliver and Paul-Shaheen challenge the paradigmatic view of the policy entrepreneur as a "singular leader … with a blueprint for action" and finds that innovation was achieved through an "internal team process of policy design" melding technical and political analysis. Using a market analogy, they describe it as "not so much the brilliant salesmanship of someone offering a finished product as it is a group assignment for product development … more like internal innovation within a large corporation than market entry by a start-up firm" (Oliver 1997, p. 746).

A growing body of research has focused on seeking to enhance the recognition of institutional factors in the MS Framework. Zohlnhöfer and Rüb (2016a, pp. 2–4) acknowledge that the MS Framework can be applied to very different contexts than that for which it was originally designed because policymaking in parliamentary democracies is changing, issues are more complex and contestable, time pressures are increasing and the role of party ideology is diminishing. Policymaking in these jurisdictions has changed and started to look less like a rational response to a defined social or economic problem. However this widening use reinforces the need for much more theoretical refinement of the MS Framework, its analytic value and its empirical applicability than has occurred to date.

This work is very promising. For instance Spohr (Zohlnhöfer 2016a, p. 251) contends that institutions "shape constellations of actors and their goals" and "channel and shape participants' behaviour, which helps to determine which solutions reach the agenda." His work merges elements from a single-theory institutionalist approach with the MS Framework to describe non-incremental change in the United Kingdom and Sweden. In these case studies, institutions permit path-departing change, for instance where increased competitive pressure, policy learning or the weakening of elites occurs. This requires a policy window to open in the Politics Stream and the use of this window by policy entrepreneurs who shape a path through clever discourse or by minimising risks of blame for unpopular new policies. Béland (2005) merges institutionalist approaches and the MS Framework by identifying the key role played by policy entrepreneurs in successfully drawing on existing repertoires to frame new policy alternatives. However he reminds us that formal institutions largely determine which actors are in a strong position to become policy entrepreneurs, and they influence the way frames affect political debates. He also contends that ideational processes can be subordinate to institutional elements, citing Schmidt's comparative study of the importance of discourse in gaining agreement for policy reform. Of note in that study, the same two single-actor systems, the United Kingdom and New Zealand, are studied (Béland 2005). Zohlnhöfer et al. (2016b) adapt the MS Framework by focusing on the need to recognise the role of institutions at the decision-making stage. They suggest that a distinctive process of coupling is added to this stage in which formal institutions may come into play in a decisive way. They add the "political entrepreneur," who operates in this stage, to the MS Framework and this person may differ from the policy entrepreneur who drove the agenda-setting phase.

The "institutional" entrepreneur model is a more recent concept in the literature. Researchers have identified actors who seek to change institutions rather than policies, looking for opportune moments to innovate and introduce new forms of governance. They carry out public mandates, combining the authority of the state with their specialised knowledge and/or other private resources such as capital or technology. They often recombine existing arrangements in innovative ways (Crouch 2005; Tuohy 2012). Buhr proposes a perspective that sees them "evolving activities at work rather than what makes unique individuals or organisations successful" (Buhr 2012, p. 1569). If their "endowment" is expertise, they must operate within the norms of a knowledge-based community (Tuohy 2012, p. 7). The risks they take relate to engaging their endowments of knowledge with current political incumbents (which may place them at risk with successor administrations). Where, in a health policy environment, entrepreneurs act from a base of professional knowledge they must "exercise their professional discretion in tension with the objectives of public authorities" (Tuohy 2012, p. 9). Crouch emphasises the recombinant features of his model, hypothesising that institutional heterogeneity facilitates innovation by presenting actors with alternative paths. Tuohy has said that in Britain, between 1990 and 2010, health service redesign had both "favoured and been accelerated by the emergence of institutional entrepreneurs" (Tuohy 2012, pp. 2–4). Institutional fragmentation, heterogeneity (and loose coupling of resources in the environment to permit reconfiguration) and political uncertainty (created for instance by periods of major policy change) provided favourable conditions for institutional entrepreneurs. While not explicitly seeking to modify the MS Framework, it is clear that these institutionalist theorists have identified a variation on the role of policy entrepreneur of the MS Framework which could lead to its adaptation.

The research on pay-for-performance policymaking in England and New Zealand presented in this book adds new insights about the effects of formal political institutions on public policymaking which are relevant for the MS Framework. This research has tested two core hypotheses of the MS Framework: that non-incremental change occurs in conditions of ambiguity of preferences, fluidity of participation and unclear technology; and that policy entrepreneurs are required to couple the three streams at the agenda-setting stage. It has reviewed the utility of the Framework, to explain the policy change and variation observed, in tandem with the utility of single-theory approaches. Its findings offer a challenge to the assumption that conditions of ambiguity, fluidity of participation and unclear technology are necessary pre-conditions for non-incremental policy change, especially in "more orderly" parliamentary systems (Zahariadis 2003, p. 1) or that a policy entrepreneur is necessary to couple the three streams at the agenda-setting stage. The case is also made for further refinement of the MS Framework by recommending the inclusion of "Institutional context" as a sub-element of the Politics Stream and acknowledging the differing types of entrepreneurs, operating at different stages and with different goals, in the Policy Entrepreneurs element. By making these refinements, policymakers using the MS Framework will discover many more options to assist them to plan for and achieve successful non-incremental policy change.

## Notes

1. Policy community and policy network or network are used interchangeably in this book, depending usually on the preferred term used by another researcher when the concept is being discussed in relation to their work. For instance, John prefers "network," Kingdon uses "policy community" and Zahariadis uses both.

## References

Aberbach, J. D., & Christensen, T. (2001). Radical Reform in New Zealand: Crisis, Windows of Opportunity, and Rational Actors. *Public Administration, 79*(2), 403–422.

Béland, D. (2005). Ideas and Social Policy: An Institutional Perspective. *Social Policy and Administration, 39*(1), 1–18.

Buhr, K. (2012). The Inclusion of Aviation in the EU Emissions Trading Scheme: Temporal Conditions for Institutional Entrepreneurship. *Organization Studies, 33*(11), 1565–1587.

Cohen, M., March, J., & Olsen, J. (1972). A Garbage Can Model of Organisational Choice. *American Science Quarterly, 17*, 1–25.

Crouch, C. (2005). *Capitalist Diversity and Change*. Oxford: Oxford University Press.

John, P. (1998). *Analysing Public Policy*. London: Cassell.

Jones, M., Peterson, H., Pierce, J., Herweg, N., Bernal, A., Raney, H. L., et al. (2015). A River Runs Through It: A Multiple Streams Meta-review. *Policy Studies Journal, 44*(1), 13–36.

Kingdon, J. W. (2010). *Agendas, Alternatives, and Public Policies, Update Edition, with an Epilogue on Health Care*. London: Longmans.

Kusi-Ampofo, O., Church, J., Conteh, C., & Heinmiller, B. T. (2015). Resistance and Change: A Multiple Streams Apporach to Understanding Health Policymaking in Ghana. *Journal of Health Politics Policy and Law, 40*(1), 195–219.

Marsh, D., & Rhodes, R. A. W. (1992). *Policy Networks in British Government.* Oxford: Clarendon Press.

Mintrom, M., & Norman, P. (2009). Policy Entrepreneurship and Policy Change. *Policy Studies Journal, 37*(4), 649–667.

Mintrom, M., & Vergari, S. (1996). Advocacy Coalitions, Policy Entrepreneurs, and Policy Change. *Policy Studies Journal, 24*(3), 420–434.

Oliver, T. R., & Paul-Shaheen, P. (1997). Translating Ideas into Actions: Entrepreneurial Leadership in State Health Care Reforms. *Journal of Health Politics, Policy and Law, 2*(3), 721–788.

Sabatier, P. a. W. (Ed.). (2014). *Theories of the Policy Process.* New York: Westview Press.

Strand, M., & Fosse, E. (2011). Tackling Health Inequalities in Norway: Applying Linear and Non-linear Models in the Policymaking Process. *Critical Public Health, 21*(3), 373–381.

Tuohy, C. H. (2012). *Institutional Entrepreneurs and the Politics of Redesigning the Welfare State: The Case of Health Care.* New Orleans, a paper to be presented at the annual meeting of the American Political Science Association, New Orleans, Louisiana.

Zahariadis, N. (1995). Ideas, Networks, and Policy Streams: Privatization in Britain and Germany. *Policy Studies Review, 14*, 71–98.

Zahariadis, N. (2003). Ambiguity and Choice in European Public Policy. *Journal of European Public Policy, 15*(4), 514–530.

Zahariadis, N. (2007). The Multiple Streams Framework. In P. A. Sabatier (Ed.), *Theories of the Policy Process.* Boulder: Westview Press.

Zohlnhöfer, R., & Rüb, F. (Eds.) (2016a). *Decision-Making under Ambiguity and Time Constraints.* Colchester: ECPR Press.

Zohlnhöfer, R., Herweg, N., & Rüb, F. (2016b). Bringing Formal Political Institutions into the Multiple Streams Framework: An Analytical Proposal for Comparative Policy Analysis. *Journal of Comparative Policy Analysis, 18*(3), 243–256.

# CHAPTER 3

# A Comparison of the English and New Zealand General Practice Sub-Systems

**Abstract** Comparative analysis has been described as the closest social science can get to generating and testing hypotheses. Here, the history and features of the general practice sub-systems of the English and New Zealand national health services are compared and contrasting features identified in order to understand their differing processes of policymaking. Despite many similarities at their time of origin and in recent episodes of health policy reform, the two general practice systems have diverged widely in important elements. The gradual development of a single-payer state-sponsored partnership between general practitioners and the state in England is contrasted with the growth of a multi-payer system in New Zealand in which general practitioners had a fractious relationship and no formal partnership with the state.

**Keywords** History of New Zealand and English general practice • New Public Management health reforms

The general practice sub-systems of England and New Zealand differ substantially, though both countries have national health systems with many other features in common, and general practice services are delivered by independent medical practitioners. The historical legacies of the two health services, necessary for this comparison of health policymaking, are set out below. Each arose in the immediate pre- and post-World War

II period when both countries elected Labour parties with large majorities, reflecting a climate of growing support for collectivist approaches to social and economic challenges and rising public demand and need for health services. Medical professional interests were well organised and sought opportunities to be part of health policy development (Lovell-Smith 1966).

## THE ENGLISH STORY

In 1945 England elected a Labour government with skilled and determined politicians of working-class origin and a mandate for major social change, financed on a collectivist basis (Tuohy 1999; Ham 2004; Klein 2006). There was a shared sense, developed over several years by both state actors and health professionals, of the need for a state-sponsored plan for a comprehensive range of health services, to be free at point of use (Tuohy 1999, p. 38; Klein 2006). Public opinion supported a 1942 report by William Beveridge that recommended the establishment of a national health service among other widespread reforms to the system of social welfare.

The incoming government proposed a capitated, free and universal service, though it initially sought to employ doctors on salaries. The British Medical Association (BMA) fought its major battle to avoid implementation of a salaried general practice service and to engage general practitioners as independent contractors to the Department for Health. But in the process of the larger battle over terms of employment, the Secretary of State, Aneurin Bevan, established the principle that treatment would be free at the point of delivery throughout the health system and that payment would be on a capitation basis rather than fee-for-service. Bevan dealt separately with the interests of general practitioners and specialists during the negotiations. Dividing the profession by offering improved conditions to specialists, the Secretary was able to win agreement to the proposed legislation from the profession overall, carried on the votes of satisfied specialists despite the concerns of general practitioners.

Doctors retained their clinical autonomy, including the right to prescribe medicines and treat as they saw fit. But in England a system of single-payer state-sponsored "hierarchical corporatism" ensued (Tuohy 1999), otherwise described as the "politics of the double bed" (Klein 1990), in which the bureaucracy and the profession, both specialists and general practitioners, established strong organisational forms and a track record of partnership to support the interdependent relationship between the state and doctors. Doctors were formally represented and held effective veto rights at each level of the new hierarchy.

## THE NEW ZEALAND STORY

The difficult birth of the general practice element of New Zealand's national health service between 1935 and 1948 is set out by various writers (Lovell-Smith 1966; Hanson 1980; Bolitho 1984; Belgrave 1985; Hay 1989; Fougere 1993; Belich 1996, 2001; King 2003). In 1935, New Zealand's Labour party had been elected in a landslide victory. The idea of a free universal health service, although it had been Labour party policy since 1919, broke relatively new public policy ground. The new government began a three-year process of consultation with stakeholders and exploratory research, including seeking advice from the BMA (which represented New Zealand doctors), to determine how it would be implemented.

The medical profession rapidly emerged as a powerful stakeholder in the policy process. Doctors were, by 1935, among the highest paid professionals in the land. On average their salaries were equal to those of the top civil servants at that time (Bolitho 1984). Ninety-two per cent of New Zealand's doctors were members of the BMA in 1927 (Belgrave 1985, p. 360) and were organised into regional and provincial divisions, each with its own executive and standing committee. Business was "conducted in a painstakingly democratic way, and only in very difficult situations is any Committee of Council given authority to act without approval of the Divisions" (Lovell-Smith 1966).

With Labour's election in 1935, and faced with a proposal for a universal capitated tax-payer-funded free health-care system, doctors resolved to oppose this on various grounds, including: that it was unnecessary to introduce financial support except to the poorest patients; the greater need was for public health and preventive services and the state should concentrate its effort and resource upon this area of need; that free treatment would result in overuse of services by patients; and perhaps greatest of all, that doctors feared state control of medical practice and socialised medicine. The profession was opposed to the scheme not only on economic grounds but from an "inherent and deep conservatism" and fear of state control of their work (Hanson 1980). Other mechanisms were at work too. Fougere contends that the profession had a less hierarchical structure in New Zealand than in England at that time and that leaders of the profession were more likely to be general practitioners with additional training or specialism (Wilkes 1984, p. 79). For instance, three-quarters of the Committee negotiating with the government about general practice services were specialist practitioners (general practitioners who also had a specialism in an area of medicine). Specialists on the committee had a clear interest in sustaining their lucrative practice with wealthy patients. (This institutional feature meant that the profession was unified in a way not seen in England where specialists had separate streams of representation to government and ministers could exploit the different interests between these two tiers of medicine.) In New Zealand a remarkable degree of unity and unanimity persisted among the profession for the long years of dispute with the government, eventually bringing a significant victory by changing the method of payment originally proposed and allowing the right to charge patients additional payments.

The Social Security Bill in early 1938 set out very high-level promises for free health care for all and generous remuneration to doctors, based on capitation, not salaried service. Though it was designed by a medical colleague, Dr McMillan, a Labour Member of Parliament, 828 of 913 doctors opposed the proposed legislation. In particular, they objected to its universality. The proposed legislation was publicly announced and formed the basis of the health manifesto for Labour in that year's general election. Labour was re-elected, its share of the vote increasing to 56 per cent. The government implemented the Act in April 1939, disregarding the overwhelming opposition of doctors. Following protracted negotiation, the general practice service provision initially provided, in 1941, for a contract for patients to present to their doctor whereby the doctor could charge his costs to the new Social Security Fund (into which citizens had been contributing a share of their tax payments since 1938). It was based upon a generous capitated payment and allowances for travel and other procedures. The proposed legislation was confined to payment arrangements and made no attempt to limit clinical freedom, making contracts voluntary. General practitioners overwhelmingly boycotted the offers of government contracts for their services and continued to charge patients in full for their services.

Widespread Friendly Society enrolment by citizens seeking affordable health care had ceased, and income for general practitoners, which had been primarily guaranteed by Friendly Society income and rapidly rising, dropped sharply by 1941 as a result (Belgrave 1985, p. 180). Patients began sending their invoices for treatment to the government. Faced with declining support and an election in 1941, the government tabled a further Bill offering, this time a very generous fee-for-service payment arrangement, but prohibiting co-payments and effectively making the new arrangements compulsory. This was passed without the support of the BMA. Patients could then claim a refund of their fees from the Ministry of Health. Some doctors commenced the practice of receiving "token" payments from patients in addition to their basic fee, which was of dubious legality, but endorsed by the Ministry. Incomes soared again, surpassing those of specialists (Lovell-Smith 1966, p. 156). However, the profession had lost its unity on the issue of payment processes and methods of payment proliferated.

Finally in 1949, following a review of the operation of the service, and shortly before the Labour government faced yet another election, legislation was enacted to settle upon the mechanism of a direct fee-for-service claim on the Social Security Fund by the doctor and the provisions prohibiting co-payments were repealed. This was "a victory for the medical profession and demonstrated the strength of its bargaining power ... [and] effectively sounded the death knell of the free general practitioner service aimed at and legislated for in 1938" (Hanson 1980, pp. 124–5). The implementation of the Social Security Act which established New Zealand's national health system resulted in the state's responsibility being "tempered by compromises between the government of the day and an organised and assertive medical profession" (OECD 1994, p. 227).

## KEY DIFFERENCES

In England the National Health Service Act of 1946 made consultation costs free at the point of care and all patients were registered with a general practice. Until 2004 general practitioners were directly contracted to provide services and paid from a mixture of capitation, fees-for-service, allowances and infrastructural funding in the general practice contract with the National Health Service (NHS). In many respects general practitioners had a great deal of freedom about where and how they organised their work, what care they delivered, and they largely owned their premises. In 1966 a key change to their contractual conditions was negotiated to include reimbursement of expenses of practice staff and opportunities to invest in premises and equipment. The core of the contractual provisions for general practices was an allowance to cover practice expenses, to which weighted capitation funding for patients was added and, in many cases, fees for the delivery of particular services. Though general practitioners were independent contractors of the NHS, they were entirely dependent upon it for the income to maintain themselves and their practices, which included access to pension schemes and other terms and conditions of employment.

In New Zealand the General Medical Services scheme introduced in 1941 provided a universal subsidy for general practitioner services (the patient health benefit), though general practitioners ultimately retained the right to charge patients (Smith 2010, p. 27). There was no contract-for-service between an individual practitioner and a public funder for the services delivered to patients in New Zealand, and patient registers were voluntary and incomplete in 2000. The subsidy for visits to a general practitioner, originally covering about 75 per cent of the total fee, dropped to an average of 20–30 per cent of the total fee by 1986. Together with government funding, patient co-payments and private insurance reimbursement of general practices fees, general practice services funding has several small pools. No funder established monopsonistic influence. The extensive out-of-pocket payments in New Zealand primary health care creates barriers to access for some sectors of the population (Brown 1997; Crampton 2000; Tuohy 2004; Croxson 2009). General practitioner interest groups have resisted attempts to control their fees and to introduce contracts (Hay 1989; Davis 2000, p. 203).

## SHARED HISTORY OF NEW PUBLIC MANAGEMENT-BASED HEALTH REFORMS DURING 1990s

England and New Zealand developed shared concerns in the 1980s about rising costs of health care. Both countries also identified inequities in access to high quality health care and in differing life expectancy and health outcomes for different groups within their population. Reform evolved in the 1990s by strengthening the hand of third-party payers through more active forms of purchasing and the introduction of competition in quasi-markets within health systems (OECD 1994; Tuohy 1999, pp. 19, 26; WHO 2000, pp. 13–14). Episodes of health policymaking which deliberately excluded the medical profession to minimise perceived conflicts of interest in policy development occurred in both countries, such as the 1990 NHS and Community Care Act (Tuohy 1999, p. 70) in England and the 1993 Health and Disability Services Act in New Zealand (Crampton 2000; Laugesen 2000). These active purchasing strategies can be summarised as use of performance measurement, contracting, market-type mechanisms and customer orientation to manage public or publicly funded services. In England the widespread use of performance indicators had commenced in 1983, focused on hospital services and designed to monitor the performance of the new Regional Health Authorities (Pollitt 2010).

In New Zealand this focus was introduced in 1989 with contractual frameworks that specified targets, plans and funding levels and defined the obligations of both parties between the 14 Area Health Boards and the Minister of Health (Boston 1991, p. 281). Both countries implemented bold system-level reforms in which the pace and scope of change in each system has been called "big bang" reform (Tuohy 1999; Fougere 2001; Tenbensel 2008). The extent of the convergence, or shared policymaking approaches, in health system reform and neo-liberal social and economic reforms taken by both countries is often noted in the literature (OECD 1994; Marsh 2001). Tuohy comments that in Britain "sweeping change in the public politics governing the [health] decision-making system [was] enacted and implemented. More modest versions of the British reforms took place in Sweden and New Zealand" (Tuohy 1999, p. 4). In 2004 the OECD noted that "while most countries have focused on the hospital sector, both Britain and New Zealand have experimented with using primary care doctors as purchasers" (OECD 2004, p. 57). Both countries adopted contractual frameworks, in particular budget-holding, as the preferred method to encourage general practitioners to adopt funder goals such as greater efficiencies, improved coordination of care and improved quality and responsiveness of care. It is in this context that some small-scale local fund-holding, pay-for-performance and budget-holding initiatives began to be trialled in both countries (Spooner 2000; Fougere 2001), but in general practice settings which had widely different accountability relationships between state funders and the profession.

The shared pathway of health service reform from 1991 is summarised in the Table 3.1:

**Table 3.1** General practice systems: England and New Zealand—key features and changes during reform period

| *England—pre-1990* | *New Zealand—pre-1990* |
|---|---|
| Services comprehensive, free at point of use, universal | Services comprehensive, subject to co-payments, universal |
| Singular governance and ownership structure. All GPs self-employed, with individual contracts with NHS, supported by public funding for premises, infrastructure, pension provisions and so on. BMA has sole bargaining rights for all GPs | Hybrid forms of ownership and governance: some GPs self-employed in privately owned practices, some GPs in non-profit owned practices, small number in special areas employed by state. No contracts for general medical services between GPs and state |
| Contracts for government funding:<br>– Base salary for practice costs<br>– Capitation based on number of patients (50 per cent of income)<br>– Fees for certain procedures | Income from fees-for-service from patients and government subsidies<br>(Patient co-payments and subsidy for targeted patients ("health benefit")) |
| Gatekeepers to specialist services | Gatekeepers to specialist services |
| All patients enrol with a GP—free choice of GP | Most patients register with a GP—free choice of GP |
| Public funding by single demand-driven centrally set prospective budget (Department of Health) | Public funding by multiple demand-driven centrally set and administered prospective budgets (Ministry of Health, ACC, other) |
| **1990–1997** | **1990–1999** |
| More explicit GP contract-for-service | GP funding transferred to contract-based with primary care organisations over time. However, GPs still largely received income on fee-for-service basis. |
| | Health purchasing authorities formed to identify local needs and trial new services. Māori and community-oriented services established. |
| | Corporate or meso health organisations formed (IPAs and others) to negotiate contracts for services on behalf of individual practices in many areas. |
| | A process for reviewing the reasonableness of fee increases introduced. |
| | Funding for primary and secondary care integrated in regional purchaser budgets Increased focus on public health |
| GP fund-holding for secondary care available for large practices (based on weighted capitation budget) from 1993 | Some GP budget management agreements for pharmaceuticals and laboratory testing negotiated between regional purchasers and general practice organisations |

*(continued)*

## Table 3.1 (continued)

| England—pre-1990 | New Zealand—pre-1990 |
| --- | --- |
| | "Free" GP care for under-six-year-olds implemented |
| Competitive internal market for health services encouraged | Competitive public/private market for health services encouraged |
| | Attempt to define core services |
| Patient's Charter | Focus on patients' needs/preferences |
| National, centralised quality initiatives (National Institute for Health and Care Excellence, Commission for Health Improvement) | IPA-initiated Guidelines production Guidelines Group established |
| **Post-1997** | **Post-1999** |
| Personal Medical Service contracts available for meeting local needs | |
| Intermediate organisations of Primary Care Groups assumed commissioning for all secondary services, replacing budget-holding | Intermediate organisations (PHOs) established to commission and manage primary care services |
| | Integrated purchaser/provider function for health services established in 21 regions |
| | Primary care funding moves to capitation basis through contracts between DHBs and PHOs (but GPs still received income on fee-for service basis initially) |
| | GP fees review structure re-established to manage excessive fee increases |
| | All patients required to enrol in a PHO via a GP |
| | Expanded amount and basis of entitlement for health benefits |
| Focus on public health services and importance of prevention and population-based health services | Focus on public health services and importance of prevention and population-based health services |

## REFERENCES

Belgrave, M. (1985). *"Medical Men" and "Lady Doctors": The Making of a New Zealand Profession 1867–1941.* PhD thesis, Victoria University of Wellington, New Zealand.

Belich, J. (1996). *Making Peoples.* Auckland: Allen Lane.

Belich, J. (2001). *Paradise Reforged.* Auckland: Allen Lane.

Bolitho, D. G. (1984). Some Financial and Medico-Political Aspects of the New Zealand Medical Profession's Reaction to the Introduction of Social Security. *New Zealand Journal of Health, 18*(1), 34–49.

Boston, J., Martin, J., Pallot, J., & Walsh, P. (Eds.). (1991). *Reshaping the State*. Auckland: Oxford University Press.

Brown, M. C., & Crampton, P. (1997). New Zealand Policy Strategies Concerning the Funding of General Practitioner Care. *Health Policy, 41*, 87–104.

Crampton, P. (2000). Policies for General Practice. In P. Davis & T. Ashton (Eds.), *Health and Public Policy in New Zealand*. Auckland: Oxford University Press.

Croxson, B., Smith, J., & Cumming, J. (2009). *Patient Fees as a Metaphor for So Much More in New Zealand's Primary Health Care System*. Wellington: Health Services Research Centre, Victoria University of Wellington.

Davis, P., & Ashton, T. (2000). *Health Policy and Public Policy in New Zealand*. Auckland: Oxford University Press.

Fougere, G. (1993). Struggling for Control: The State and the Medical Profession in New Zealand. In F. W. Hafferty & J. B. McKinlay (Eds.), *The Changing Medical Profession*. Oxford: Oxford University Press.

Fougere, G. (2001). Transforming Health Sectors: New Logics of Organizing in the New Zeland Health System. *Social Science and Medicine, 52*, 1233–1242.

Ham, C. (2004). *Health Policy in Britain*. Basingstoke: Palgrave Macmillan.

Hanson, E. (1980). *The Politics of Social Security*. Wellington: Auckland University Press.

Hay, I. (1989). *The Caring Commodity*. Wellington: Oxford University Press.

King, M. (2003). *The Penguin History of New Zealand*. Auckland: Penguin Books.

Klein, R. (1990). The State and the Profession: The Politics of the Double Bed. *BMJ, 301*, 700–702.

Klein, R. (2006). *The New Politics of the NHS*. Abingdon: Radcliffe Publishing.

Laugesen, M. (2000). The Institutional Context. In P. Davis & T. Ashton (Eds.), *Health and Public Policy in New Zealand*. Auckland: Oxford University Press.

Lovell-Smith, J. B. (1966). *The New Zealand Doctor and the Welfare State*. Auckland: Blackwood and Janet Paul.

Marsh, D., Richards, D., & Smith, M. J. (2001). *Changing Patterns of Governance in the United Kingdom*. Basingstoke: Palgrave Macmillan.

OECD. (1994). *The Reform of Health Care Systems*. Paris: OECD.

OECD. (2004). *Towards High Performing Health Systems*. Paris: OECD.

Pollitt, C., Harrison, S., Dowswell, G., Jerak-Zuiderent, S., & Bal, R. (2010). Performance Regimes in Health Care: Institutions, Critical Junctures and the Logic of Escalation in England and the Netherlands. *Evaluation, 16*(1), 13–29.

Smith, J., Mays, N., Ovenden, C., Cumming, J., McDonald, J., & Boston, J. (2010). *Managing Mixed Financing of Privately Owned Providers in the Public Interest*. Wellington: Institute of Policy Studies.

Spooner, A., Chapple, A., & Roland, M. (2000). The PRICCE Project, National Primary Care Research and Development Centre, University of Manchester.

Tenbensel, T. (2008). How Do Governments Steer Health Policy? A Comparison of Canadian and New Zealand Approaches to Cost Control and Primary Health Care Reform. *Journal of Comparative Policy Analysis: Research and Practice, 10*(4), 347–363.

Tuohy, C. H. (1999). *Accidental Logics.* Oxford: Oxford University Press.

Tuohy, C. H., Flood, C. M., & Stabile, M. (2004). How Does Private Finance Affect Health Care Systems? Marshalling the Evidence from OECD Nations. *Journal of Health Politics, Policy and Law, 29*(3), 359–396.

WHO. (2000). *The World Health Report 2000.* Geneva: World Health Organisation.

Wilkes, C., & Shirley, I. (1984). *In the Public Interest.* Auckland: Benton Ross.

# CHAPTER 4

# England: Context and the Quality and Outcomes Framework

**Abstract** England's Quality and Outcomes Framework is one of the most ambitious, large-scale pay-for-performance schemes ever designed for general practitioners. Negotiated between the British Medical Association and the state between 2001 and 2004, the detailed story of its design is told in rich detail, often in the voices of the policymakers. Drawing on insights from 12 qualitative interviews with participating or proximate policymakers in England, the context and background to the policymaking is set out and the transformative intentions of policymakers revealed. The reader is allowed to see who was involved, what was done, how it was done and how it was implemented. Significant barriers which threatened the process, and enablers which supported it, are described and discussed.

**Keywords** Quality and Outcomes Framework • Pay-for-performance • Principle-based negotiation • Clinical autonomy

## BACKGROUND

Before the 1997 election, England's Labour Party set out health policy proposals to improve collaboration between the hospital and primary care sectors, tie funding of services to best practice as validated by clinical audit (or "getting patients a better service more quickly") and change the two-tier fundholding system in general practice (Mandelson 1996, pp. 148–49). After the election, the new government focused on policy initiatives designed to replace competition with collaboration and partnership. It established Primary Care Groups and Trusts. The Groups were general practitioner-led advisory bodies in the first instance, evolving to Trusts which could commission care and provide community services. They had a strong population-based and health-promotion-oriented purpose and a clear mandate to ensure good clinical governance of medical practice.

## THE NHS PLAN 2000

In 2000 the government published its second major policy plan for health services, the NHS Plan (Secretary of State for Health 2000), with proposals for a new national pay-for-performance programme for general practitioners as part of a new General Medical Services contract. The purpose was, according to Prime Minister Tony Blair, "all about trying to introduce systems where the money spent was linked to performance and where the service user was in the driving seat" (Blair 2010). He had dramatically announced new investment in health in January 2000 in an interview on BBC Television's *Breakfast with Frost*, promising to bring expenditure on Britain's NHS up to the European Union average of 8 per cent of GDP (Seldon 2007, p. 69) from 5.7 per cent. However, as a quid pro quo for this huge new investment, the Prime Minister also set out five challenges: "partnerships, performance, professions, patient care and prevention" (Secretary of State for Health 2000). Reforms would include "using incentives to kick-start the modernization … to increase the quality of health care and to see the customer driving progress throughout the NHS" (Seldon 2007, p. 44). The NHS Plan also contained a commitment to reduce health inequalities. The newly elected Labour government had established a Minister for Public Health and commissioned a report on health inequalities to "put reducing health inequalities at the heart of tackling the root causes of ill health to create a fairer society and to reduce the costs associated with ill health" (Comptroller and Auditor General 2010). Pay-for-performance was central to the NHS Plan, which involved "a complete redesign of the terms and conditions for working in the NHS" according to the newly appointed Junior Minister, John Hutton, who was put in charge of negotiating the new General Medical Services contract at the time.

## A Challenge to Centralism

The Prime Minister acknowledged Labour was continuing efforts of the previous government of "breaking down centralized and monolithic structures, about focusing on the developing tastes of consumers, about ending old demarcations in professions" (Blair 2010, p. 262). A process of "constructive discomfort" was implemented which put pressure on the relationship "between the British state and medical profession for most of the post war period, with the medical profession taking responsibility for the quality and allocation of publicly-funded care, in return for professional autonomy and the absence of intrusive state regulation" (Stevens 2004). Stevens identifies three strategies: providing support for providers, top-down imposition of standards and targets and applying countervailing pressure on providers from strategies such as competition between different suppliers, which, in primary care, included enhanced patient choice of provider "be they public, private or not-for-profit ... Private diagnostics and primary care out-of-hours services are next." It also included aligned provider incentives ("GPs' new contracts will allow them to earn around a third more, linked to markers of quality"). There was recognition that if working conditions and support for health professionals were improved, they could be relied upon to "do the right thing" by patients. Government, acting as proxy for consumers, would set targets and national standards for the quality and outcomes of health services, publicise these and, where necessary, intervene to ensure performance improved.

The Prime Minister wanted improved support for providers and plurality of supply. "GPs had a complete monopoly. Competition, even in the event of a hopeless service, was literally banned.... Health care systems in which there was mixed public/private provision, or which at least demanded some individual commitment and gave some individual choice, did best ... surely it must be possible to combine equity and efficiency" (Blair 2010, p. 215, 319). At his speech to the Labour Party Conference in 2001 the Prime Minister claimed that "without reform, more money and pay won't succeed" (Seldon 2007, p. 69). The strategy of pay-for-performance was therefore championed at the highest level of the core executive. A strongly motivated team of health ministers had been appointed to implement the changes. The Secretary of State for Health appointed in 1999 was a "modernizer" by contrast to his "traditionalist" predecessor (Ham 2004) and was, in Blair's words, "fully simpatico with the direction of change" (Blair 2010, p. 264). John Hutton had the task to manage the re-negotiation of three NHS contracts: the General Medical Services contract, the Consultants contract and the contract for other NHS staff (called the Agenda for Change). These contract negotiations were seen by him as a key part of the implementation of the NHS strategy as a whole.

## WHO WAS INVOLVED

A participant recalls the reaction from 10 Downing Street when, on a day in the middle of the 2001 election campaign, the BMA gave:

> an ultimatum that said if they didn't get a new GP contract they would contemplate downing tools and stopping serving NHS patients, resigning from the NHS ... [Downing Street] believed ... given there was this independent system of pay review bodies that a substantial earnings uplift was legitimate and so one way or another [they] were likely to have to pay more for GP services. So then the question ... was ... to use this opportunity to pivot to a ... deal in which rather than simply seeing increased pay [it was possible to] get something in return for it. That was the intellectual genesis of the new contract and the QOF.

The Prime Minister also decided on the same day to contract out the negotiation of the new contract to the NHS Confederation (the membership body for all organisations that commission and provide NHS services). Dr. John Chisholm, Chair of the BMA's General Practitioners Committee, initially wondered if the decision to outsource the negotiations was, by depriving the BMA of the direct bargaining relationship with ministers, "punishment for the insubordination" of the campaign run by the BMA for better working conditions during the 2001 election. In England, the relationship between the medical profession and the state was one of mutual dependency, described by Klein as the "politics of the double bed" (Klein 1990), in which the profession ran the NHS and rationed its scarce resources but was entirely dependent upon the state, as a monopoly employer, for income and resources. The BMA would reasonably have feared that this special relationship was now over.

Ministers chose Mr Mike Farrar, having had a successful record in leadership roles in the Department of Health, as the Chairman for the Confederation team of negotiators. John Hutton thought of this new Chairman as someone who was very strong, experienced, knew primary care and was trusted for his basic judgement about how these contracts could be renegotiated, and his judgement about the mood around the negotiating table. John Chisholm reports that the BMA liked the choice of the new Chairman. "We got on well with [him] basically because of his palpable honesty, really. He was a pleasure to do business with even when he was giving tough messages [and] would focus on the problems not the person."

The Chairman first recruited a team. Dr Tony Snell, a veteran of pay-for-performance in general practice who had led a scheme called the Primary Care Clinical Effectiveness (PRICCE) project in East Kent for over four years, was recruited. Others were either well known to the Chairman or were Chief Executives of Primary Care Trusts. The decision to outsource the negotiations was cosmetic in essence. Hutton recalls that "I wasn't in the detailed around-the-table discussions but you know I was practically in the room so this idea that it was at arm's length ... I think very few people saw that as reality." A thorough and strict selection process for team members included vetting for experience in negotiation by experts in negotiation skills development who also delivered principle-based negotiation training to the selected team.

The BMA team was formed from members of its General Practitioners Committee, selected by that Committee. The BMA at the time represented 141,000 doctors in the United Kingdom and has long had a highly democratic structure. The BMA, and thus the General Practitioners Committee, is recognised by the health departments in national negotiations for NHS general practitioners (BMA 2013). It has sole bargaining rights for all NHS general practitioners. The BMA team of doctors included those who had years of experience and training in industrial negotiation between them. In addition, the team had a trade union negotiator and expert advisers including a lawyer, a health economist, a pension expert and actuary and an innovations expert. The team had a limited mandate and was described by a participant as "actually very weak in that they are regularly re-elected, their membership is capable of kicking them out ... and they put their negotiated positions to votes of all the membership which effectively ties the hands of the negotiators."

Maintaining the support of BMA members during the process was a challenge. The negotiators did not have the same level of trust from their mandate-givers enjoyed by the Confederation team. At times it seemed to negotiators that a deal had been reached only to have the BMA come back and say their members would not live with it. Confederation team members went to lengths on one occasion to support the BMA negotiators in presenting the final framework for ratification to the representatives of Local Medical Committees of the BMA.

Civil servants had a largely observer status at all meetings of the Plenary (the whole negotiating team meeting). During the negotiations a team of academic advisers was recruited to offer independent expert evidence about suitable clinical indicators for the Quality and Outcomes Framework (QOF) and establish rigorous standards to test each indicator for suitability. A forceful presence, their rigorous tests and role as interlocutors for the evidence-based process of decision-making clearly helped to mediate and submerge the overt interests of any particular party. Without them, it is unlikely that the scope and quantity of indicators which were eventually included in the QOF could have been agreed in such a relatively short time frame.

Members of different teams had known one another for years in some cases. Seven of the eleven participants in the direct negotiations over the QOF were medical professionals. Almost all were practising general practitioners and there were professional connections between members of the team of academic advisers and many of the doctors on the teams. With the exception of the politicians and the Confederation Chair, this was indeed largely a policy design by general practitioners for general practitioners.

## WHAT WAS DONE

John Hutton held overall responsibility for the contract negotiations, with the intention to achieve all the top-line messages. The top line included a need to

> shift more of the money into prevention, more public health [and] more resources to be paid to general practitioners on the back of results rather than just per capita [and] to address was workforce-related issues ... The theory then was that there was a chronic workforce shortage in primary care that a more generous contract would begin to address. It wasn't just a question of resources—better outcomes, better pay and so on—there was also this work/life balance. Under the old contract a lot of the GPs felt they were being flogged to death almost.

He recognised these recruitment and retention issues within general practice had a serious equity perspective:

We were chronically under-doctored in many parts of the country. We were also looking very much at this question of equity of provision in primary care. Over 50–60 years what had happened here ... a lot of the resource had gravitated to the better-off areas. We never had a problem recruiting general practitioners in the home counties, the nicer parts of Britain. But we could not find a way of getting general practitioners to work in those areas which had the greatest health needs because they couldn't make the sort of money and the work was harder.

General practitioners' fees and allowances regulations were described by Mr Farrar as set out in an "old Red Book [which] was hugely complex ... with massive amounts of money being spent without any sense of what we got back for it in terms of value, patient benefits, health outcomes, information. It was bureaucratic, often fraudulent, paid practitioners to have high list sizes and promoted entirely reactive general medical care." This meant that a major transformation was required to meet ministers' expectations of rewarding quality and health outcomes.

John Hutton strongly identified with elements of an agenda for resolving access and quality concerns in the under-doctored areas of Britain. Inequity of health service access and health outcomes was common in the North West of England. A participant confirms that he saw Hutton as seeking to achieve a "culture change so the system worked more for patients and less for clinicians in areas such as access times, reflections of patients' expectations in general practice and so on."

The expectations of No. 10 were, according to a participant, "what would be the most help to the public to get out of these changes in working relationships? What is wrong at the moment, what needs to be fixed?" Ultimately the outcome of the negotiations can be seen to present a set of clear priorities of No. 10 for responsive services as well as improvements in equity of access and outcomes.

This keenness for responsiveness resulted in the removal of out-of-hours care from the contract and the transfer of the responsibility for its delivery to intermediate organisations which would source it from other private or non-profit providers. This achieved two goals—the top-line requirement of the BMA for improved working conditions for doctors, as they could opt out of the delivery of out-of-hours care, and the goal of introducing competition into primary care services through the contracting of these and other services to new entrants to the primary care market.

The priorities for No. 10 were seen by participants as linked to the concern to preserve electoral support for a tax-payer funded universal health service. Some thought the service was "undersupplying appropriate care, causing long waits for routine surgeries" (Stevens 2004, p. 37) and inviting increasing adverse media commentary that compared the NHS negatively with allegedly better health services in continental Europe. This gave the government a "mandate to act as a proxy for the consumer using four powerful new hierarchical levers mostly absent from the previous Conservative government's 1991 health reforms": national standards and targets, inspection and regulation, published performance information and direct intervention in the event of poor performance (Stevens 2004, p. 40).

The BMA wanted a new contract for general practice that would give them their share of the new health funding. Their campaign for a new contract was strongly reinforced by a survey of general practitioners which showed that 97 per cent of responding practitioners said too much was being asked of them. Pension reform, the removal of the requirement for out-of-hours work and improved pay were bottom lines for the BMA. They readily agreed that a pay-for-performance mechanism could form a major part of a new contract. One participant believes "that [the BMA] had agreed to move into this territory [of pay-for-performance] without much fuss because they thought they could shape it in a way that didn't require a major shift of focus for general practitioners to new areas of work."

Even had this not been the case, it was hard for the BMA to resist the strong expectations of the Secretary of State for Health about pay-for-performance. A participant saw him as insistent that "there would be no pay rise for work already being done." He had a "bloody-minded determination for performance pay." Others describe the goal as "something for something," meaning to make a significant part of the payment to doctors contingent on quality targets being achieved. John Chisholm also says,

> the [BMA's 2001] national survey would have given some comfort to the idea that actually general practitioners did want to see rules for quality.... [The team] wouldn't have been courageous enough to have galloped off in that direction without some kind of mandate.

However, they would agree only to standards which reflected appropriate clinical performance, not political imperatives. For instance, it was believed they would resist any access standards which did not have a basis in clinical care even though they might have been asked for by patients. Targets, if they were introduced, would need to be appropriately weighted.

Both parties sought a large scheme. Government leaders believed that the success of pay-for-performance schemes like the Primary Care Clinical Effectiveness project (PRICCE) in East Kent had demonstrated the effectiveness of rewarding quality and justified a scheme with as many indicators as could be agreed. For the BMA, a larger scheme made more money available to their members. A participant believed that the pre-eminent role for the BMA in its relationship with government would be placed under serious threat if they could not broker a popular and lucrative national deal for their members.

## How It Was Done

Hutton, the Junior Minister, knew that the Prime Minister also wanted a consensus-based agreement with the BMA. He describes how:

> the previous government tried and failed and then imposed an agreement on the BMA. I can quite understand why ... [they] might have done that ... I was very reluctant to get to that point ... An imposed agreement never is going to last the test of time, not in our kind of society where people are in trade unions, there are negotiation processes, they want to be treated properly and respectfully and this is a very well-developed vested-interest group, the BMA, a very powerful group, so imposed agreement can never survive.

One of the participants describes the flawed logic of imposed settlements:

> You could do lots of dreadful things ... like in the 1990 contract and you could ... change the contract without agreement but it ultimately didn't work. People would vote with their feet and those drivers eventually forced [government] to come back and negotiate.

John Hutton led the process. He established clarity about the negotiating strategy for the team, described as "what was wanted, the top and bottom lines." This was achieved at an early point through his request for a session with the Chair, Departmental officials and academics from the National Primary Care Research and Development Centre in Manchester. This was a key moment in the design process according to one participant. "It established the framework, key issues, absolutes/desirables/not bothereds."

For the negotiators, it was important that they understood exactly what Hutton expected of the negotiations. Mr Farrar told the Minister "early on that if anyone puts a cigarette paper between you and me we are in real trouble. You need to have absolute confidence in me." Mr Farrar had "a clear understanding of what I wanted to do.... Our starting point was what was going on in the NHS which had impressed, ... [that we could] build into this contract".

The major model of a quality framework considered) by the Sub Group, PRICCE, was a voluntary quality improvement scheme implemented in East Kent in England in 1988 to improve chronic disease management. People involved in PRICCE later became key to the development of the QOF. PRICCE offered £3000 in advance to each enrolled general practitioner who could meet the entire set of targets for the clinical care of 13 chronic conditions as demonstrated by post-payment audit verification. The evaluation of PRICCE reports:

> the main motivation for doctors ... was to improve patient care. Many practices invested significantly more than the resources they were given. Key motivators for this were the alignment ... with the doctors' own professional values and the autonomy given to health professionals in how they achieved the targets ... [D]espite the considerable increase in workload required, involvement in PRICCE) was associated with increased morale among primary care staff. (Spooner, p. 3)

The Confederation team undertook, for the first time, the same type of negotiation training which had for many years been the standard curriculum in the BMA, being principle-based negotiation. Participants from both sides attest to the difference this training made to the conduct of the negotiations. Mr Farrar says:

> It was huge ... previously with the BMA when neither side were properly trained ... it was dreadful—there was banging of tables ... they did not quite walk out but nearly. Training meant we took a break and parties regrouped. This was a simple technique but avoided much grandstanding. The great value was we went through the same training programme so used the common language, common techniques. It really was a big boost for us.

John Chisholm describes principle-based negotiation as follows:

> Positional bargaining is not quite forbidden but it is not the approach you should use ... identifying your objectives, the other side's objectives in relation to that particular issue, trying to understand their position, trying to decide how far you are prepared to move.... In general, you are supposed to come at a negotiating issue in an honest way.

A government participant says: "We were trying to strengthen our hand … [by] thinking strategically … how we could look at the overarching goals that united us, then work through the framework as constructive and consultative as possible."

A participant describes it thus:

> It was very different from anything I had done before. It was quite formal. There was calling of time out, which I had not seen before. Sometimes this was quite helpful. I couldn't always work out what was going on and it allowed us to discuss how to facilitate getting an outcome.

One of the participants comments that the five Confederation team members, all either Primary Care Trust or Health Authority senior staff, were "people who knew how to trade, to negotiate; they … had the skills which you needed. Nobody could say they sent in some soft hearted pussy cat to negotiate with the BMA." Mr Farrar was seen as having exceptional negotiation skills: the participant further comments:

> If you look at good negotiators versus bad … [he] had most of those features in the quantities you expect: probing skills, revisiting skills, number of ideas per cubic metre, different ways of getting to yes, trade and bargain versus war and attack, use of humour … negotiation is not about victor and vanquished, it is about trading and coming to a wise agreement.

Participants from all sides of the process acknowledged Mr Farrar's role in facilitating this complex set of negotiations in an almost uniformly positive way. He describes some of these strategies: "We worked hard and put effort into the social bit … we tried to get people together in the evenings. You can often get agreement in that context which you cannot do around a negotiating table."

## IMPLEMENTATION

The Framework could not be implemented without designing a major new information-gathering software application suitable for installation in every general practice, which came to be known as the Quality Management Advisory System (QMAS). Having designed an indicator, a participant describes how "then we had to go on and work out how you would verify it. A whole raft of decisions and negotiations over IT was done," the participant recalls.

You started with the criteria but then you moved on to what are the standards going to be and then what are the exclusion criteria going to be and
how are you going to measure it and assess it and have somebody go out and
have a look at it. What about the IT … how were you going to deal with
confidentiality…. It was out of that discussion that we had on the one side
the practice-based system where you can look at the names and we can
search to find which patients, and you have QMAS which can't.

The data had to be extractable from the databases in each general practice,
which presented significant practical problems. Many different suppliers
provided computer systems for general practice and a small number of
practices were not computerised. Departmental officials worked with the
Connecting for Health IT team over 26 weeks to design a platform to
extract the data. Mr Farrar recalls, "These were potential show stoppers
but in each case the BMA was persuaded to allow them to proceed because
otherwise they would have lost the whole deal" and "we just crashed
through that." In the event a "high-trust" system for monitoring and
reporting achievements against targets was introduced, along with a provision for independent audit, so that general practices could be funded for
their achievements against the QOF.

By February 2003 Mr Farrar was able to write to the BMA Chair, sum-
marising the details of the new contract and attaching the 68-page document "Investing in General Practice—The New General Medical Services
Contract" for his members to consider and vote on. A negotiator recalls,
"At the end [the BMA] took it to [the membership] and there was a much
more vigorous 'no' campaign [than during earlier membership ballots on
the interim framework] but even then 70 percent supported it." It was
accepted in June 2003.

Practices were given a year to prepare for the new Framework.
Participation in the Framework was voluntary. In England 99 per cent of
practices signed up immediately and within a year they were demonstrating an average achievement of 91.3 per cent of the expected targets.

BARRIERS AND ENABLERS OF THE POLICYMAKING PROCESS

*Redistribution of General Practice Resources*

The pay-for-performance programme was one part of a wider strategy, set
out in the NHS Plan, to achieve reductions in health outcome inequalities
by increasing access to general practice services and incentivising best

practice preventive health care, but this strategic goal nearly derailed the negotiation of the contract. Negotiators had to improve the distribution of general practice funding and services according to health needs. Proposed allocations had been modelled on unrepresentative practice data; when presented to the membership of the BMA, in John Chisholm's words, "there was an absolute bloody riot in the profession and in the General Practitioners Committee ... and a series of demands for change in the detail of the contract." For many practices their guaranteed income (without payments for quality achievements) would actually go down.

[P]art of the reason for overspending on the Framework is that the department reallocated funding initially assigned to fund the Framework to the global sum (the per capita amount per practice which was not conditional upon performance), in order to fund a new Minimum Practice Income Guarantee (MPIG). It therefore revised its predictions of achievement under the QOF. Following implementation, Framework achievements exceeded those revised estimates. The overspend in the first three years was 9.4 percent more than provisioned. (Comptroller and Auditor General 2008)

Related to the equity issue were well-documented workforce supply and distribution issues within general practice. A participant confirms that "it was harder to attract new doctors to go to general practice." Another comments,

it was terrible being in general practice in 2002. It was awful, it was haemorrhaging people and at the time the government cared: we had to put something in place that restored morale and recruitment and if we could do something about implementing chronic disease management to a higher level that would also be very good.

The right to withdraw from provision of out-of-hours service and the appropriate sum to be deducted from practice income if the practice opted out of provision of that service was part of this deal. However this backfired: Hutton concludes that "the loss of the Saturday surgeries [because of the after-hours settlement] was an error from our point of view."

Notwithstanding this consequence, politicians also got improvements in organisational standards, such as measuring patient satisfaction and access times for appointments, through the contract. A participant reports, "Ministers were trying to achieve not just a level of outcome but a culture change so the systems worked more for patients and less for clinicians." The focus on non-clinical indicators was a major area of discord, and consequently a significant achievement for the Confederation team.

### Balancing Funder Interests and Clinical Autonomy

The key funder interests which the new contract needed to reflect were public health goals, greater patient responsiveness and pay-for-performance approaches to quality improvement. The "public health agenda was a 'must-have' for ministers ... [a public health issue such as] obesity was a close-fought issue," according to one participant. Managing the risks of obesity was a cherished target for politicians but sceptically viewed by those charged with finding the evidence-based case for a general practice-based intervention. A commentator agrees that work on the NHS Plan showed how "poor we were in clinical outcomes compared to other countries. And we were particularly poor in heart disease and cancer".

A participant confirms that

> ... the Framework is great ... it has helped push up in the back half of the roughly normal distribution curve ... got public health stuff in there up to a point (we are still quite light on the public health stuff) ... the main focus was on some of the chronic disease areas.... The real benefit from the QOF was the standardisation of the bottom half of the performance spectrum.

This did, however, raise the issue of whether incentives would work too well according to another participant:

> there is ample evidence of a very strong behavioural response by health professionals including primary care doctors to financial incentives ... you have got to calibrate them incredibly carefully and the best forum for doing that is probably not a high profile political negotiation between the medical profession and government.

### Shaping Patterns of Interaction Between the State and Interest Groups

Several new patterns of interaction can be seen in this negotiation: the new governance role for intermediate organisations, the Primary Care Trust (PCT in England and the Primary Care Organisations elsewhere) as holders of the contract; the explicit consideration of the expectations of patients and their needs for access to general practice services; and principle-based negotiation as a pattern of interaction which was intended to encourage a sharing of goals rather than a contest for victory.

For the first time in the history of contract negotiations between the state and the BMA, this was "a contract for primary care services between a commissioner and an organisation, the PCT," with the intent to encourage "chronic disease management locally" among other objectives, as well as a negotiation over terms and conditions of work for practitioners.

Another new challenge was how to deal with the different interests of the BMA and patients. This presented a test for Labour: John Hutton says,

> you form a government and take responsibility for public services—when you think about the NHS we have this horrible habit of thinking just about the unions.... You always have to think about the patients, the consumer. That's the discipline, it's a tough one—the Tories found it easier than [Labour] for the first few years.

The negotiation of the contract generally and the QOF in particular had a flavour of consensus and partnership. Hutton "wanted consensus … agreement that would stand the test of time … imposed agreement can never survive" and believed "it was an important political process to get right."

Participants report a clear sense of the competing interests of the BMA on the one hand to minimise the challenge of the new targets and of the politicians through their departmental officials, on the other hand to extend the targets that would stretch general practice to improved levels of clinical quality. John Chisholm describes the process of negotiation:

> In terms of the level of challenge, on many indicators the GPC would have been wanting a lower range and the NHS Confederation and the Department of Health would have been wanting a higher range. … [Not] in relation to every indicator but that would have been the pattern. So … you did find that there was a bit of positional bargaining; however, … one was trying to avoid that. In general, people were starting off in different places and through negotiation and compromise they moved towards each other.

Mr Farrar says "The BMA knew our intention over time was to make it stretchy and we knew they would make this hard." An official concurs, describing BMA representatives as saying "You can have that much quality or that much quality—have you got that much money or that much money?"

Another says:

> They [the BMA] had some degree of acting as a union but they weren't
> totally doing that, they were also interested in patient care and quality and
> doing what they could get away with and if it was going to be really hard it
> was going to be costly for someone, which was fair enough. I don't think
> any one group felt they had won. It was a good negotiation from that point
> of view.

The Confederation team, however, had credibility with the BMA and
inspired their trust. BMA negotiators saw it as "a watershed in the way the
government does business with the BMA." Dr Snell notes that that "there
was a huge amount of distrust between the BMA, the union and the government negotiators which is why externals were brought in ... who didn't
carry the baggage that the department had."

Both parties mobilised public opinion. When the BMA threatened to
strike during an election campaign the atmosphere for the negotiations
heated up. However, the use of the media was a double-edged sword,
exposing the provisions of the contract to public view. As another participant comments, "When I look back to the past and then look at how the
GPs are now perceived I see that there is a high profile in the media and
the question 'Why aren't they open when I need them?' can now be
asked." Hutton believes that "The BMA will never again be able to parade
the argument that GPs are fundamentally underpaid ... there is no time of
day for that argument now." Another reports that "The Daily Mail has put
the overpayment of doctors in the public domain and haven't said it was
reversed" [by subsequent QOF negotiations in later years].

Structures and institutions also added pressure. According to one par-
ticipant, "The General Practitioners Committee was worried that if agree-
ment couldn't be reached government would impose or default to the
Personal Medical Services contract which was locally agreed ... [then] the
Committee would lose its mandate as a nationally representative body."
This is echoed by another participant:

> [the BMA] "were quite strongly motivated to get an attractive new contract
> structure ... to retain their negotiating influence ... So that was one of the
> other tools the government had in its negotiating armoury." Another sug-
> gests that "a lot of this was driven by the BMA scared about the incursions
> of local contracting."

The scheme had been thoroughly discussed among the BMA's general practitioners. One participant says:

> We did two sets of road-shows … they were very cynical and quite angry, but in the end we had a vote and the vast majority thought it was OK. There was a very strong "no" campaign but in the end their votes were not much— they were voting on the interim some way through the negotiations to touch base to see how it would go.

## SOLVING THE TECHNICAL CHALLENGES

### *Choice of Indicators*

The use of incentives, according to one participant,

> gave no cause for doubt or political concern … because actually GPs were already subject to a series of incentives…. [S]ince the 1990 contract the question was, "are the incentives aligned right and are we getting bangs for the buck?" … [I]n primary care, the focus was very much on chronic disease management.

The scope and speed with which the QOF was designed owes much to the legacy of the 1990 contract and the first term of the Labour government which developed national service frameworks for many of the clinical domains incentivised in the QOF.

The early days of the Quality Sub Group were fraught with tension and conflict as participants began to debate the way in which a set of indicators might be chosen and targets set for achievement in the new contract. However, once its membership had been expanded to include the academic team of expert advisers and the BMA Chair, there was surprisingly little discord between the Confederation and BMA representatives in the Quality Sub Group over the selection of the set of 146 indictors from the literally hundreds collected for consideration by the academic team.

One participant says that the experience was arduous: "the experts had been through all the schemes they could find…. [T]he only summative assessment was PRICCE." As to the atmosphere, this participant says, "in the negotiation it felt like a practice meeting … we thought the patients were going to benefit … we were negotiating this in order to achieve patient benefit…. [T]hat was genuinely what we were trying to do."

Another agrees these were "discussions rather than negotiations. The government people were very well informed. It was between peers ... [with] very much a shared purpose."

The Junior Minister, Hutton, is clear that the BMA "got the QOF to focus on things that they were by and large already doing." Another points to the "steady move from the 1990s onwards to seek to draw back the veil on the variation that exists in quality and performance in the delivery of care ... and the fact that GPs were already subject to a series of incentives." Indeed, "to start producing new criteria and standards was virtually impossible ... we went with what we had rather than producing new," says another participant. Another participant agrees that "everything was there—that was how a big scheme was done so quickly."

There was a developing acceptance by general practitioners, according to John Chisholm, "that some sort of quality assurance of their continued competence to practice was the right thing to do." A commentator confirms, "It wasn't suddenly something that was plucked out of the air and thrown into a culture that hadn't changed for years."

### Obtaining Access to Data

Data issues were identified and needed to be resolved repeatedly throughout the process of design. As described earlier, the most famous data problem arose as a consequence of incomplete practice data used to develop the model for allocation of funding to practices, causing a reduced core income for many practices. However, MPIG was designed within four days to provide protection from loss of income. Money was provisioned from the total available for the contract. This crisis attracted a high level of collaborative damage control from all the negotiating parties.

This was probably the worst moment in what Hutton describes as "the inevitable bumpy ride ... rough patches ... unexpected downsides" of the contract negotiation. He describes how "it all went belly up about ... MPIG ... and [the Secretary of State] rang and said what the ... hell is going on."

Mr Farrar agrees:

> It put us on the back foot very much. You have situations where a practice has to get twice as many pounds per head but get an equal amount of QOF points. This was particularly a concern for me with its impact on redistribution and the opportunity for the practices in the poorer areas to be supported. However, on an international level the ratio of 2:1 funding for

richest as against poorest practices is very good—it is usually 16:1 or some similar large number.

The money for MPIG was withdrawn from that earmarked for quality payments but by that time the Framework and the price per point had been ratified by the membership of the BMA and could not be renegotiated. Mr Farrar confirms:

> The only way we could do that [present a feasible total cost of contract] was to moderate our expectation of achievement. So, where we had anticipated 850 (of 1050 available points being achieved on average per practice) we then said, well ok we will [anticipate] 750—that made the numbers stack up. If we had realized this earlier we would have had a much wiser negotiation.... [I]t caught [us] on the hop and the moral of the story was [we] did not have the finance team in [our] team ... and we had come adrift.

In fact, there were several different estimates of likely achievement, ranging from 650 by one participant to 750 by the Confederation negotiators of QOF to the confident expectation of some others of the BMA team that their members would average 950.

For John Hutton,

> The biggest thing we got wrong was estimating the risk.... [W]e thought that about 70 percent of practices would score the maximum QOF points and it turned out to be 95 percent and that caused a significant amount of financial pressure in the NHS.

The media seized on these commentaries as did Opposition politicians and even some Labour politicians, criticising the failure to set a baseline performance measure of quality before implementing the QOF, so that the true extent of lift in quality could be assessed against the price paid for it.

By contrast, obtaining access to practice-level data to ensure that achievements against targets in the QOF could be tracked and points earned was relatively straightforward. Mr Farrar describes this process:

> I negotiated a deal where GPs could retain ownership of their IT but all software had to be compatible. No. 10 advised that they wanted GPs to control their IT. This meant some GPs could opt out of data collection. I thought this could be handled differently. These were potential show stoppers but in each case the BMA was persuaded to allow them to proceed because otherwise they would have lost the whole deal.

### Testing the Model

The literature suggests that pay-for-performance schemes should be trialled to avoid design flaws which might have unintended consequences. The Minister was never invited to consider trialling the contract before implementation and did not request this, according to a participant. Mr Farrar comments:

> Because PRICCE was so relevant we could see how it was going to behave. We also built in a review process so we set up a QOF review team and the principles were that this would be revisited every year; … we knew we would have got something wrong … we have to be clever enough not to be stupid and lock ourselves in. So rather than go for piloting it we set in a process [for] an ongoing review.

John Chisholm concurs for different reasons with the decision not to pilot.

> Well there is a long history about piloting. One wants evidence-based practice right across the public sector … but on the other hand I identify with the frustration that ministers and civil servants must sometimes feel and have certainly seen times in the past when the call for piloting is used as a delaying tactic; … the negotiations were more protracted than anticipated…. There was enormous pressure from general practice about why haven't we got it and we want it now! So the idea that we could then have said "that's it, and we are now going to pilot it in the Northern region for a couple of years"— we would have been strung up. There was a need to push on and do it.

The high expectations of ministers and the profession and the urgency of time also pressured the Confederation team. A participant admits that he "was one of the people pushing the negotiating team to go further, do more, try harder" in an environment where the "GP magazine [was] whipping up GP grass roots opinion and their ability to recall their negotiators." This prevented piloting of the points for the QOF to obtain more accurate predictions of achievements.

However, the agreement that indicators could be reviewed and replaced or adjusted over the years was an insurance against possible negative impacts of these technical difficulties or unintended consequences. A participant explains that "QOF has evolved as we thought it would. We never thought that QOF was going to be fixed in time but the public health agenda moves on and we will get more ambitious, I hope, as time moves on." Mr Farrar confirms:

> Since the original QOF there have been a number of changes—kidney disease introduced after three years. That has been phenomenal in diagnosing about 3% of the population with kidney disease not previously diagnosed because general practitioners weren't incentivised to go out and find it.

The BMA achieved a form of insurance against negative impacts, too. One element of the QOF which attracted criticism was the provision that practitioners could "exception report" or remove a patient from the denominator for a standard (if patients did not attend for review or if there was a contra-indication for the prescribing of a medicine), and that the upper standard for achievement of targets was 90 per cent of patients. For the BMA, exception reporting was an important provision. John Chisholm confirms that "indeed one of [the BMA's] lasting concerns was the lack of exception reporting ... for target payments for immunisation and cervical cytology [in the 1990 contract] because here informed dissent is not allowed.... We lost that argument."

However, there was evidence in the literature presented by the expert advisers that this provision could be gamed. General practitioners could seek to maximise their performance against targets by exempting patients inappropriately. The Framework set the standard for maximum points for achievement of a target when an intervention was used with 90 per cent of patients. This seemed to some commentators—and certainly to commentators in the popular and academic media afterwards—to further erode the rigour of the QOF. Mr Farrar says:

> One of my regrets is the doubling up effect of the exception reporting and the threshold provisions. We were probably over-generous about allowing the 10 percent exception because this allowed practices to give up on the hardest patients. The model was based on PRICCE but in retrospect it would be easier to have said that there were [sic] a lower level of points for up to 90 percent and higher points for the last 10 percent, thus encouraging practices to work really hard to get the gains for their resistant patients, but for the same all-up costs.

In fact, evaluations demonstrated that this risk of practices giving up on the hardest patients did not occur (Audit Commission 2011).

## Evaluations and Reviews of the Scheme

In the three years following the implementation of the new contract, Doran reports that having begun the decade in near crisis, by 2009 primary care in Britain excelled in information technology, access, chronic care management, performance review and patient satisfaction (Doran 2010). The number of general practitioners rose by 15 per cent and the vacancy rate fell from 3.1 per cent to 0.8 per cent, though the distribution of general practitioners between affluent and more deprived areas became less equitable as new practitioners chose to practice in more affluent areas. Morale, as measured by the BMA survey in 2008, showed improvements, though half continued to report low morale.

In 2008 the National Audit Office published "NHS Pay Modernisation: New Contracts for General Practice Services in England" and concluded that recruitment and retention and skill mix within general practice had improved, though the contract had not increased productivity (i.e. the Department expected returns which had greater benefit than the amount of money put into the new contract). The Office found that it was too early to tell whether quality had improved but found increased flexibility of PCTs to increase the breadth of services for patients. While there had not been a significant increase in patient satisfaction, the Audit Office considered the contract had assisted in the development of an entrepreneurial culture, with PCTs able to contract services to competing private sector providers to meet local needs. General practitioner satisfaction increased initially with the implementation of the contract but by 2008 had not been maintained.

In a report for the National Institute for Health Research Delivery and Organisation programme published in 2010, McDonald et al. find that the QOF achieved accelerated improvements in quality for two of three chronic conditions; however, once targets were reached the improvement in care of these patients slowed, and declined for some conditions not linked to incentives. However, the variation in care quality related to deprivation in general medical practice reduced over time. McDonald concludes that this suggests that QOF has the potential to make a substantial contribution to the reduction of inequalities in the delivery of care related to area deprivation (McDonald 2010).

The Final Report of the National Institute for Health Research programme confirmed statistically significant associations between higher levels of achievement on QOF clinical indicators for coronary heart disease, hypertension, congestive heart failure, diabetes and chronic obstructive pulmonary disease, and reductions in rates of ambulatory care hospital admissions (Dixon 2010, p. 121). A study in 2009 found that for most indicators that can be assessed, QOF incentive payments were likely to be a cost-effective use of resources even if only modest improvements in care were achieved (Walker 2010). In deprived areas, QOF achievement reflecting the performance of general practice was outweighed by wider social determinants of health, leading the evaluators to conclude that insufficient incentives for practices in deprived areas existed to identify and manage patients to prevent admission to hospital. The report hypothesised that exception reporting and targets below 100 per cent, taken together, may have undermined the incentives for practices in these areas to actively search out such patients for follow-up. It concluded that "it may prove challenging to shift the focus of general practice from providing medical services to taking responsibility for population health and reducing health inequalities" (Dixon 2010, p. 20).

The QOF has been considerably analysed by researchers in England, in addition to official evaluations of the scheme. One impact has been the development of an extensive database of general practice activities that is now available to researchers interested in primary health care questions. One study of the impact of withdrawal of indicators in subsequent iterations of the QOF has found that levels of performance generally remained stable, and concluded that health benefits from incentive schemes can potentially be increased by periodically replacing existing indicators with new ones relating to alternative aspects of care. However, the indicators removed remained directly or partly incentivised by other indicators in the QOF, so this research is therefore subject to the caveat that full withdrawal of incentives may deliver different results (Kontopantelis 2014).

Regarding patient views about QOF, in a study of exception reporting of patients to investigate whether this had been informed dissent, it was found that this was relatively infrequent, suggesting that the incentivised activities were broadly acceptable to patients (Doran 2012). A minority of patients in a later qualitative study noticed and appreciated the questions their general practices were now asking, such as about smoking and weight, which were driven by evidence-based prompts in the electronic medical records of patients developed for the implementation of the QOF (Hannon 2012).

Another study explored whether the QOF led to the neglect of activities not included in the scheme (based on a longitudinal analysis of 42 activities of which 19 were not included in the scheme). It found that by 2006–07, improvements for 14 incentivised activities were significant, reached a plateau quickly but remained higher than predicted by pre-incentive trends, whereas the non-incentivised indicators achievement rates were significantly below those predicted by pre-incentive trends by 2006–07 (Doran 2011).

In 2009 a new way of developing indicators for the QOF was introduced, involving piloting with a testing protocol. A study of the results of this protocol found that there was considerable value for money in pre-testing the implementation issues relating to acceptability and unintended consequences as well as technical reliability and feasibility of indicators (Campbell 2011).

By 2016, analysts were assessing its benefits primarily in new sources of population data on major conditions, modest improvements in quality of care for chronic diseases in the QOF and reduced inequalities between deprived and less deprived areas. This has led to recommendations to reduce payments and increase patient-centred quality measures (Steele 2016).

## References

Audit Commission. (2011). *Paying GPs to Improve Quality*. London: Audit Commission.

Blair, T. (2010). *A Journey*. London: Hutchinson.

British Medical Association. (2013). How We Work. Retrieved 19 May 2013. https://www.bma.org.uk/about-us/how-we-work

Campbell, S., Kontopantelis, E., Hannon, K., Burke, M., Barber, A., & Lester, H. (2011). Framework and Indicator Testing Protocol for Developing and Piloting Quality Indicators for the UK Quality and Outcomes Framework. *BMC Family Practice, 12,* 85.

Comptroller and Auditor General. (2008). *NHS Pay Modernisation: New Contracts for General Practice Services in England*. London: National Audit Office.

Comptroller and Auditor General. (2010). *Tackling Inequalities in Life Expectancy in Areas with the Worst Health and Deprivation*. London: National Audit Office.

Dixon, A., Khachatryan, A., Wallace, A., Peckham, S., Boyce, T., & Gillam, S. (2010). *The Quality and Outcomes Framework (QOF): Does It Reduce Health Inequalities?* Final Report. London: National Institute for Health Research.

Doran, T., & Roland, M. (2010). Lessons from Major Initiatives to Improve Primary Care in the United Kingdom. *Health Affairs, 29*(5), 1023–1029.

Doran, T., Kontopantelis, E., Valderas, J., Campbell, S., Roland, M., Salisbury, C., et al. (2011). Effect of Financial Incentives on Incentivised and Non-incentivised Clinical Activities: Longitudinal Analysis of Data from the UK Quality and Outcomes Framework. *BMJ, 342*, d3590.

Doran, T., Kontopantelis, E., Fullwood, C., Lester, H., Valderas, J., & Campbell, S. (2012). Exempting Dissenting Patients from Pay for Performance Schemes: Retrospective Analysis of Exception Reporting in the UK Quality and Outcomes Framework. *BMJ, 344*, e2405.

Ham, C. (2004). *Health Policy in Britain*. Basingstoke: Palgrave Macmillan.

Hannon, K., Lester, H., & Campbell, S. (2012). Patients' View of Pay for Performance in Primary Care: A Qualitative Study. *British Journal of General Practice, 62*, e322–e328.

Klein, R. (1990). The State and the Profession: The Politics of the Double Bed. *BMJ, 301*, 700–702.

Kontopantelis, E., Springate, D., Reeves, D., Ashroft, D., Valdeas, J., & Doran, T. (2014). Withdrawing Performance Indicators: Retrospective Analysis of General Practice Performance under UK Quality and Outcomes Framework. *BMJ, 348*, g330.

Mandelson, P., & Liddle, R. (1996). *The Blair Revolution*. London: Faber and Faber Limited.

McDonald, R., Cheraghi-Sohi, S., Tickle, M., Roland, M., Doran, T., Campbell, S., et al. (2010). The *Impact of Incentives on the Behaviour and Performance of Primary Care Professionals*. Report for the National Institute for Health Research Service Delivery and Organisation Programme Manchester, National Institute for Health Research Service Delivery and Organisation Programme.

Secretary of State for Health. (2000). The NHS Plan. Health, The Stationery Office.

Seldon, A. (2007). *Blair Unbound*. London: Pocket Books.

Steele, N., & Shekelle, P. (2016). After 12 Years, Where Next for QOF? *BMJ, 354*(i4103). https://doi.org/10.1136/bmj.i4103.

Stevens, S. (2004). Reform Strategies for the English NHS. *Health Affairs, 23*(3), 37–44.

Walker, S., Mason, A., Claxton, K., Cookson, R., Fenwick, E., Fleetcroft, R., et al. (2010, May). Value for Money and the Quality and Outcomes Framework in Primary Care in the UK NHS. *British Journal of General Practice, 60*(574), e213–e220.

# CHAPTER 5

# Utility of Kingdon's Framework: Policymaking in England

**Abstract** Kingdon's Multiple Streams Framework hypothesises that policy change happens when policymakers' preferences are ambiguous, there is fluid participation and unclear technology, and entrepreneurs are able to exploit this uncertainty in brief windows. These hypotheses are challenged in this case study of policymaking in England between 2001 and 2004. Both the Multiple Streams Framework and five single-approach theories of policy change (institutions, groups, rational choice, ideas and socio-economic circumstances) are tested against the case study evidence of design of a pay-for-performance scheme. Kingdon's Framework is the most useful approach but fails to encourage recognition of the powerful institutional and interest group factors at work. Amendments to the Framework to reflect ownership and governance arrangements and the role of state-appointed institutional entrepreneurs are recommended.

**Keywords** Multiple Streams Framework • Historical antecedents • Institutionalism • Parliamentary systems • Rational choice drivers • Bargaining

© The Author(s) 2018
V. Smith, *Bargaining Power*,
https://doi.org/10.1007/978-981-10-7602-2_5

## NON-INCREMENTAL CHANGE IN CONDITIONS OF AMBIGUITY, FLUID PARTICIPATION AND UNCLEAR TECHNOLOGY?

The first questions the MS Framework invites are whether this policymaking episode meets Kingdon's predictions about when incremental and non-incremental change occurs and the conditions under which these types of change are likely to occur. The pay-for-performance policymaking process in England was non-incremental change in Kingdon's definition and was achieved in a planned, top-down process of policymaking. Politicians had clear plans to achieve a major change in the way the NHS worked through pay-for-performance. The policy idea appeared quickly on the policy agenda, was widely understood and accepted and was quickly implemented. However, Kingdon's predicted conditions for non-incremental change are less apparent. Instead of ambiguity, there was a clearly set policy goal to introduce pay-for-performance. Instead of fluid participation, the participants at all stages of the policymaking were carefully selected and admitted to a closed and orderly process. Only a small number of aspects of the technology to implement pay-for-performance (relating to data collection) were unclear. The decision to introduce pay-for-performance into the new General Medical Services contract was taken by the Prime Minister, the Secretary of State and the Prime Minister's adviser on health policy at a discussion between themselves during the election campaign. It was, however, a process to which carefully selected participants were admitted, and the description of the process by participants suggests little ambiguity of policy preferences. While the technology of design and implementation debated at that discussion contained some innovative elements, such as the use of Confederation negotiators instead of civil servants, in most respects the planned approach was one of business as usual for ministers and their colleagues from the BMA.

The process of alternative selection, as conducted between the government and the BMA, occurred in a closely managed process with rigorously controlled participation and rules of engagement between the negotiating teams. It was based upon a completely unambiguous policy preference for pay-for-performance and had clear and existing technology for implementation (i.e., through the new contract for General Medical Services), though strongly contending interests needed to be managed during this phase.

## PROBLEMS STREAM

The major items in the Problems Stream that policymakers observed in 2001 were public concerns about access to and quality of health services (see Politics Stream, below, for more detail) and general practitioners' concerns about their terms and conditions of work. Quality in this case also means patient responsiveness.

Policymakers in this episode found out about these problems through a combination of electoral, media, policy community and interest group activity. The indicators included polling during the election campaign showing public concerns about the quality of service offered by the NHS, surveys showing 48 per cent of practitioners were planning to retire before the age of 60, increasing shortages of doctors in areas of socio-economic deprivation, and studies showing increasing variation in the quality of care, especially in areas of socio-economic deprivation. Focusing events included the BMA threat during the election campaign to go on strike and with-draw their services from NHS work, raising the level of need for a new contract, and exposure of poor health service delivery in media commentary during the election campaign ("Winston's attack [on Labour's handling of the NHS] ... was now leading the news.... Milburn did well doing the rounds but it was all pretty difficult" (Campbell 2012, p. 208)). Positive feedback which encouraged policymakers to respond to the problems through pay-for-performance approaches was also available through ministers hearing about and inspecting successful programmes such as PRICCE. A summative evaluation of this scheme was available and suggested a workable model.

The load of other problems on policymakers' agendas at the time was not a barrier, as the Prime Minister wished to concentrate policymaking efforts on domestic agenda items and recognised that these had been neglected in the previous term. The government had built high capacity and willingness for bold sweeping domestic policy initiatives.

In Zahariadis' view, policymaking which originates in the problem stream, as this does, will be more likely to lead to a rational approach in which the solution is consequential upon the problem identification. This is borne out by the evidence in the case study. A rational top-down approach was followed, consequential to the threat of general practitioners to strike. The Prime Minister and Secretary of State utilised academic advisers to provide ideas and alternative solutions about pay-for-performance extensively as part of the contract negotiations. So the model makes an accurate prediction of this link between the type of problem and the type of policymaking followed in the case study.

## POLITICS STREAM

The MS Framework specifies that in the Politics Stream, party ideology, national mood, the attitudes of interest groups and administrative turnover will be the main considerations relating to agenda-setting.

In 2001, party ideology in the Labour Party strongly supported increased investment in the NHS and centralised approaches to the management of public services. Re-engineering public services to be more responsive to citizens as service consumers was a key policy goal of "New" Labour ideology. Polling of the national mood found that health service quality and effectiveness was a key electoral issue for voters. Its electoral salience was heightened by the attention paid to the issue of poor quality of NHS service by the media. The mood was reflected in highly critical media reports during the election campaign, exposing examples of poor quality of health services. Kingdon notes that media are often portrayed as powerful agenda-setters (Kingdon 2010, p. 57) but his research reveals that they are regarded as having an important impact on the government agenda in only 26 per cent of his interviews. Participants confirm that the media *was* important in this issue. The electoral salience of health policy was a vivid concern to the New Labour politicians and their media advisers. The BMA's strike threat, which created a risk of further immediate pressure on service levels, can be seen as carefully timed for the middle of an election campaign so they could put maximum pressure on politicians through the media. Once the decision to negotiate a new contract had been taken, the medical media, including the *British Medical Journal*, was attentive to the ongoing negotiation of the new contract. Participants on both sides of the negotiation reflect their ever-present concern about the impact which adverse media coverage may have had on their achievement of their policy goals.

The general media had less insight into the process of negotiation during the policy design phase but criticised "overpayment" of general practitioners after the impact of the scheme was apparent. This had some influence in subsequent negotiations and also affected the public reputation of the BMA and doctors generally. As future negotiations over general practice contracts occur, it will be a matter of interest to see if these perceptions of overpayment will have survived in public opinion and whether, if they have, this will influence the conduct of later negotiations in any way.

The opportunity provided by administrative or legislative turnover was a key factor in creating the need for new policy, particularly health policy. The election victory with its large majority provided the opportunity for selection of new ministers in the team who were, like the Secretary of State, "fully simpatico with the direction for change." Kingdon's MS Framework and Zahariadis' model rightly anticipates the importance of administrative turnover for the agenda-setting process. Administrative turnover is even more important in adversarial Westminster policymaking environments because of the heightened "structural interest in product differentiation and incentive to initiate [policy] changes" to garner electoral support (Steinmo 1992, p. 24), the greater level of executive autonomy a large Parliamentary majority allows and the support of a professional civil service to implement new policy in these environments.

However, the major considerations in the Politics Stream in this case study were two-fold. The first was how to deal with an institutional issue about the need to negotiate a new contract for general practitioners. The second was an interest group issue: how to respond to the threat of practitioners to strike. The first of these is not easily categorised in the Zahariadis model's sub-elements in the Politics Stream.

## POLICY STREAM

The Framework identifies value acceptability and technical feasibility (or the ease with which the chosen policy can be implemented) as they affect two elements in the Policy Stream: the policy idea and the policy community as important factors in whether a policy gets on the agenda, as well as resource adequacy. These are explored below. Zahariadis' model also specifies the importance of the level of integration of the policy community and its access to decision-makers, mode of decision-making, its size and capacity as key factors in whether policies get onto the agenda. Kingdon sees the policy community to include bureaucrats, academics and researchers, which Zahariadis expands to include analysts in think tanks, interest groups and lobby groups.

**Policy idea:** In the "soup" of ideas in the Policy Stream, pay-for-performance for primary health care was clearly present. Members of the health policy community were able to draw on recent research into the effects of pay-for-performance nationally and internationally and within the primary care sector. Its chances of selection were increased by its value acceptability to all parties as a way of incentivising changes in quality of health actions, equalising access for poorer communities and improving customer responsiveness. The mechanism for policymaking managed the risks of value-conflict by using principle-based bargaining and relationship-building tactics to soften and manage disputes. This mechanism also engaged the doctors and ensured "alignment with the doctor's own professional values and the autonomy given to health professionals in how they achieved the targets" through their active participation in the policy design process. All general practitioners affected by the negotiations were able to vote on its acceptability and a majority voted in favour.

The policy idea also had technical feasibility. In the case study evidence, antecedent policies, existing pay-for-performance schemes, extensive national service frameworks providing evidence-based quality standards and research showing how to incentivise health professional behaviour, and its risks, were all available to policymakers. Show-stopping problems such as the lack of a shared database to monitor achievements against targets were tackled willingly by both parties. Although general practitioners had various practice management systems for patient record-keeping and concerns about maintaining confidentiality of patient information, a suitable technical infrastructure to support the scheme, the QMAS, was quickly designed. Linking the scheme to the negotiation of the new General Medical Services contract provided an incentive for doctors to quickly implement the changes on a national scale. However, the importance of the collective action of doctors in debating, voting and agreeing to participate in the scheme is arguably more important than the technical process of designing the system. That practitioners had a unified representative structure to negotiate on their behalf facilitated the rapid negotiation and implementation of the scheme. So these issues of technical feasibility, though significant, were quickly overcome because both parties wanted to achieve the rapid implementation of a large-scale scheme.

The evidence indicates that resource adequacy was an enabling factor in this policymaking process. Policymakers knew a pay increase for general practitioners was inevitable and wished to make it contingent on performance. General practitioners supported pay-for-performance primarily as a vehicle to increase their pay, not in its own right as a policy idea. This means that other drivers for the willingness of practitioners and the BMA to support this policy are likely to be stronger than the idea of pay-for-performance itself. Alternative drivers are discussed in the section "Importance of rational choice drivers" later in this chapter.

**The policy community**: The integration level of the health policy community concerning general practice issues can be said to be towards the high end of the continuum in England (defined by Zahariadis as consensus-based, in which there are more frequent and more formalised contacts, characterised by bargaining or sounding out and compromise). The BMA is an example of a highly integrated policy community within the larger health policy community. Although the community experienced growing divergence of forms of practice and contracts and growing heterogeneity of interests and attitudes to particular policies, there was an effective and well-resourced mechanism to coordinate these debates. The representative mechanisms of the BMA and its General Practitioners Committee, the debating and voting framework for general practitioners and the sole mandate it held to negotiate with government on behalf of all general practitioners in a closed negotiation process gave it a robust structure for coordination of policy debates in the community.

The BMA continued to have very high levels of access to politicians. This government, like earlier Labour governments, sought constructive engagement with interest groups, in semi-corporatist arrangements, and reinstated a strongly consensus-based approach to the policymaking process (a return to the "politics of the double bed"). Debates about quality and equity of access and other key issues were readily shared through the *British Medical Journal* and the media.

Within the pay-for-performance policymaking process, collegial and friendship links and shared research interests linked members of the design team, regardless of which "side" of the negotiation process they sat on. The evidence suggests that these informal integrating links between individuals facilitated debate, resolving conflicts and building constructive relationships between all participants. To further build the level of integration of the policymaking design team there was a very careful process of selection of all participants and very restricted access for new members. A high degree of administrative capacity was also provided by both parties to support the policymaking (though not quite enough financial modelling or time was available to the Confederation team to identify and manage some risks).

This sub-element of Zahariadis' model is therefore a useful and important one for the analysis of this case study.

## POLICY WINDOW

In Zahariadis' model of the MS Framework he suggests that the character-istics of the policy window can be analysed according to its coupling logic, decision style and its institutional context. One type of logic is consequen-tial: the coupling occurs because of a compelling event. Another is doctri-nal: it occurs because of a totemic policy position held, for instance, by a newly elected administration. How the coupling proceeds will also reflect whether the decision-making style of the administration in power is bold or cautious.

In this policy window the institutional context was important. The pay-for-performance policymaking had a coupling logic which was consequen-tial on the opportunity presented by a long second term in office for the government and the demand to negotiate a new General Medical Services contract. However, it was also doctrinal in that the government's policy priority for the term was to bring major improvements to general practice services as part of a doctrinal principle of modernisation of public services in general. The decision style was bold—indeed the decision to make pay-for-performance the primary element of the new arrangements flew in the face of caveats in the literature about its risks. These opportunities com-bined to ensure that the Department could couple its readiness for bold non-incremental change with the available policy window. The negotiat-ing parties' enthusiasm for speedy delivery of a contract, combined with this boldness, resulted in some flaws in design and higher than expected costs in the short term.

This type of policy window is not a matter of chance. It appears regu-larly in adversarial Westminster jurisdictions. The electoral cycle offers a routine opportunity for political parties to review policies and refine mani-festos, and there are incentives to differentiate policies between political parties. In majoritarian unitary electoral systems, party manifestos of vic-tors can be more assured of immediate implementation and politicians and civil servants can plan this process. The civil service prepares in advance for the post-election rush to implement manifesto commitments and is adept at serving new governments neutrally and efficiently in this process. This reduces the element of unpredictability and chance in policy windows in these systems.

The addition of institutional context as a sub-element of the policy window is an important adaptation to the MS Framework.

## Policy Entrepreneurs

Kingdon and Zahariadis promote the role of actors, particularly policy entrepreneurs, as important drivers of policymaking in conditions of policymaking ambiguity. Such actors are able to manipulate events to gain support for their pet policy idea in these conditions. In their view it is this role which facilitates non-incremental change when the conditions are right. Zahariadis' expanded model suggests that the activities of policy entrepreneurs can be analysed according to three criteria: access to decision-makers, resources to influence policymaking and use of strategies (such as "framing, salami tactics, affect priming and symbols") to gain support for pet policies.

The conditions of ambiguity were not found in the pay-for-performance policymaking process. No *exogenous* policy entrepreneur could be identified during the research. However, it identified several roles played by key *endogenous* actors which clearly facilitated this non-incremental policy change. These actors needed to consider which strategies would best build support for the pay-for-performance policy. The first of these actors is the Prime Minister during the agenda-setting stage, who seized an opportunity to utilise a preferred policy. The Prime Minister used strategies such as framing for the traditional Labour supporters and the unions with the message "without reform, more money and pay won't succeed." For the public it was "the service user in the driver's seat." The Secretary of State added the mantra of "something for something" to focus the efforts of the negotiation team and this became a "symbol" of the rationale for the new contract among its designers.

The second is a small group of specially recruited actors who had roles which were developed during the alternative selection stage. These actors undertook activities which resemble descriptions of institutional and policy entrepreneurs respectively as these have been developed in recent writing. These are:

- the Chair of the Confederation team, an institutional entrepreneur who exhibited the required strategic skills to obtain agreement to the policy within the whole negotiation process of the contract; and
- the leader for the Confederation team on the Quality Sub Group, exhibiting policy entrepreneurial skills, who ensured that the key features of the scheme he implemented in East Kent, PRICCE, became the primary model for the QOF.

Mintrom and Vergari's (1996) three key attributes of discovering unful-filled needs and suggesting innovative ways to meet them, bearing repu-tational risks in uncertain situations and resolving collective action problems by assembling networks to undertake change, are exemplified in the problem-solving approach taken by the Confederation Chair during the negotiations. Mintrom's concept (Mintrom 2009, p. 656) of "insider sensibilities," or deep knowledge of relevant procedures and the local norms that serve to define acceptable behaviour, was also clearly exhibited by the Confederation Chair. He resembles, in Kingdon's terms, "people who can act as change agents by making connections across disparate groups and engaging with proximate policy-makers." He conveys a moti-vation for improving the terms and conditions of doctors and the out-comes for patients, as well as disappointment at not being able to do more in these areas. His "palpable honesty" was acknowledged by other nego-tiators and he was much admired for his techniques of constructive problem-solving.

Manipulative strategies such as framing, used by the Prime Minister in agenda-setting, are not used here. Salami tactics or tackling the problem in small slices is explicitly rejected. Openness and principle-based bargain-ing techniques were the primary strategies employed in the policymaking process.

In the Quality Sub Group, the policymaking environment was differ-ent. The Chair of the Quality Sub Group was a passionate defender of his ideas and upheld these through the rough and tumble of negotiation at all costs, in Roberts' words like "the brilliant salesmanship of someone offer-ing a finished product" (Roberts 1991), leading to the respectful acknowl-edgement of the BMA that the government negotiators were not "some soft hearted pussy cats." Other innovations were then developed to man-age the risk of negotiation break-down: the Chair of the BMA team joined the group and the Chair of the Confederation team enlisted the services of independent academic interlocutors to settle the process into a balanced and manageable debate, actively using strategies from principle-based negotiation to maintain a constructive environment of problem-solving.

Although these actors do not play the roles of policy entrepreneurs as originally described by Kingdon, they are examples of new forms of endogenous institutional and policy entrepreneur which reflect the needs in the different policymaking rhythms and risks of the Westminster setting.

## ENTREPRENEURIAL RISK-TAKING

Intrinsic to the concept of entrepreneurship is that risk will be taken in order to obtain greater reward than would be derived through more conventional or routine (and therefore less risky) processes. Risk is at the heart of Kingdon's theory that non-incremental policy change is often possible only when entrepreneurial forces are brought into play. The policy and institutional entrepreneurs identified above took risks characteristic of this entrepreneurial behaviour to a certain extent. Taken at the direction of politicians in one administration, they may render the strategies of the entrepreneur inappropriate for a successor administration. The major risks taken as part of the pay-for-performance design process are explored below:

**Public support risk**: the risk that some aspects of the negotiation might result in loss of public support. This proved to be accurate. Media commentary that an excessively generous settlement for general practitioners had been reached and the furore over the wholesale cessation of Saturday morning surgeries created public frustration and the criticism that doctors would now receive much greater pay for reduced hours of work. The Prime Minister himself was confronted by unintended consequences of the new contract when he was advised on live television that it had created an incentive to prevent booking of appointments in advance, thus reducing rather than increasing easy access and responsiveness of services to the general public.

**Design risk**: the greatest design risk taken was to retain a large share of the income under the new contract as contingent upon performance (to maximise the effect of the incentives in the new contract). As the targets proved to be easy for most practices to reach, this resulted in a better-than-budgeted performance under the performance-related pay provisions. The Auditor General's confirmation that the cost of the scheme was excessive in return for relatively poor productivity gains (Comptroller and Auditor General 2008), at least in the immediate period following the negotiation, was the consequence.

## EXPLANATORY COMPREHENSIVENESS OF KINGDON'S MS FRAMEWORK

To recap, this case study exhibits a non-incremental policymaking process which runs counter to Kingdon's predictions because it occurs in a planned, top-down way in conditions of great clarity of policy preference.

In the agenda-setting phase it has none of the features of ambiguity, fluid participation and unclear technology predicted by Kingdon to create conditions for non-incremental change. No exogenous actor using political manipulation was identified (though endogenous actors with a role to facilitate major change were deliberately recruited by the administration to achieve this result). The pay-for-performance policy in the alternative selection phase was developed in a rational and top-down way, but utilising negotiation. Kingdon acknowledges in further reflections on his original framework that a "government might generate its own agenda and can be at least somewhat autonomous" (Kingdon 2010, p. 230). Zahariadis confirms that in the Problems Stream, rational approaches that are consequential upon the identification of problems may occur. He invites us to specify the conditions under which and the ways in which policymaking works from the top down. This case study shows an example of policymaking in these conditions. The key conditions here were a clear electoral mandate for change, a large parliamentary majority, a bold parliamentary leader with able colleagues and civil servants to assist him, an interest group keen to negotiate a change in their members' conditions and well-studied policy antecedents to provide confidence of the policy idea's feasibility.

There is thus a partial fit between Kingdon's Framework as elaborated by Zahariadis and the complex processes observed in the case study of the design of the QOF. On some large and important predictive theoretical positions, such as the link between chance and non-incremental change, the MS Framework has not been accurate. In many other aspects of the policymaking process there is a strong resonance between the components of the model developed by Zahariadis and the empirical evidence of how this policymaking process unfolded.

## OTHER DRIVERS OF POLICYMAKING PROCESSES

Other key drivers not as visible in the MS Framework are set out below.

### *The Importance of Historical Antecedents*

The scope and speed with which the QOF was designed clearly owes much to the historical antecedents of the policy. Existing paths, largely arising in the 1990 General Medical Services contract, could be trodden in the design of the new policy. England and Scotland had well-developed

clinical standards for practices, with professionally led guidelines development and practice accreditation which were well-accepted by general practitioners. Kingdon acknowledges that in the alternative selection phase of
policymaking, civil servants may propose policies they have been working
on in the past and use a process of "softening up" (Kingdon 2010, p. 214).
He notes that officials will also utilise feedback about existing policies to
create new ones but in the alternative selection phase rather than the
agenda-setting phase. He acknowledges the idea of "spill over" or "estab-
lishing a principle." This captures the phenomenon that a change in
another arena of policymaking or a previous experience of policymaking
which sets a precedent of some kind will make it easier to achieve the same
sort of policymaking in the new arena. These concepts of "softening up"
and "spill over" do not capture the importance of the role of historical
antecedents (that the evidence shows laid reliable foundations for the policymaking) nor the strong momentum that drove the grand and ambitious
scale of the pay-for-performance scheme achieved in the English policymaking episode. There is a case for including these sub-elements as part of
Zahariadis' model to ensure they are considered in policy analysis using
the framework.

### Institutional and Structural Features

Kingdon's Framework and Zahariadis' model remain muted on the impact
underpinning structural features may have on the process of agenda-
setting and alternative selection, such as the relative ease with which a
Westminster majoritarian and unitary governing system can undertake
non-incremental policymaking by contrast with federal systems or those
with a separation of powers. An institutionalist approach to understanding
policymaking would look first to these features to explain patterns of policymaking. The ways in which England's governing system affected the
policymaking process differently from Kingdon's predicted patterns have
been set out above. These indicate that Westminster governing systems
seeking to implement non-incremental policy change can succeed without
having exogenous actors using political manipulation to drive such policy
change. This suggests that the Zahariadis model, if it is to be more appli-
cable to Westminster systems of this type, needs some amendment in addition to the recognition of institutional context as an important sub-element
of the policy window element.

The institutional landscape for a system or sub-system (such as the health system or the general practice sub-system) and the way that this might structure the relationships between the state and interest group actors has also been shown to be an important factor in a policy design process. The general practice sub-system landscape included a singular form of ownership for general practice with:

- a semi-corporatist working relationship between the BMA and the state;
- a single-payer financing arrangement for general practice;
- a single national contract between most general practitioners and the Department;
- a centralised structure for health policymaking;
- a single national representative body for general practice.

The analysis of the evidence shows that, together with the policy antecedents, these features enabled a context of bargaining and negotiation—"something for something"—which greatly facilitated the speed, scale and scope of the policymaking on a national basis. The legitimating of a single general practice organisation as representative of practitioners was crucial to the successful and rapid conduct of the design and implementation process. This also facilitated the design and implementation of the QMAS to resolve information management difficulties.

### Importance of Rational Choice Drivers

The case study evidence shows that individual actors were important in the successful design of the pay-for-performance policy, acting in entrepreneurial ways. There are also some clear rational choice drivers that can be identified at the heart of this policymaking process, operating both individually and collectively. The major driver was the prospect of greater rewards. The first example of this is the way general practitioners collectively chose a guaranteed practice income and improved terms and conditions over retention of absolute clinical autonomy. Second, individual practitioners avidly implemented the pay-for-performance programme, a voluntary scheme, in their own practices to secure this increased income. Third, the BMA chose to negotiate a lucrative contract mindful of the need to preserve its sole bargaining mandate. All these drivers were important to achieving the rapid design and implementation of this policymaking process.

It should be noted that other rational choice drivers were present too. They included support for quality indicators of practice and doing what was best for patients. From the economic point of view, "physicians do not only try to maximise income and minimise workload. Their utility function consists of other non-price elements such as ethical restraints, professional standards which may dilute or even completely remove incentives for physicians to provide ineffective care" (Saltman 2005, p. 191).

The existence of an institutional framework for bargaining and negotiation enabled the profession to make these choices to trade some clinical autonomy for greater income. So the opportunity for bargaining and negotiation, or the use of rational choice drivers, was facilitated by the institutional features of this general practice sub-system. Government negotiators respected and facilitated these institutional processes during the negotiation phase. To anticipate the analysis in the New Zealand case study, it will show a clear difference, having multiple forms of ownership and governance within general practice, multiple general practice organisations and a less integrated policy community, which gave policymakers fewer institutional features which could be used to facilitate the process of policy design and implementation.

## DOES THE ZAHARIADIS MODEL ENCOURAGE CONSIDERATION OF THESE FACTORS?

The set of sub-elements in the Zahariadis model, while recognising the importance of interest group views and the character of the policy network in which interest groups operate, does not invite sufficient consideration of institutional interest group factors such as the positional advantage conferred on the BMA with its right to hold sole bargaining rights for all general practitioners. Nor does it invite consideration of institutional factors such as the ownership and governance arrangements for health services which gave positional advantage to the state actors in this situation. These factors had a significant influence on the relative strength of different interests and actors in the policymaking process. The evidence shows that these two factors in the political stream—the mandate and resources of the BMA and the responsibilities and legal powers of the Department of Health—were vital sub-elements in the policymaking process. The sub-element relating to policy entrepreneurs does not reflect the possibility that these actors may be actively sought out and engaged by state actors to champion particular policies or governance frameworks as part of the policymaking process.

## REFERENCES

Campbell, A. (2012). *Power & Responsibility 1999–2001*. London: Arrow Books.

Comptroller and Auditor General. (2008). *NHS Pay Modernisation: New Contracts for General Practice Services in England*. London: National Audit Office.

Kingdon, J. W. (2010). *Agendas, Alternatives, and Public Policies, Update Edition, with an Epilogue on Health Care*. London: Longmans.

Mintrom, M., & Norman, P. (2009). Policy Entrepreneurship and Policy Change. *Policy Studies Journal, 37*(4), 649–667.

Mintrom, M., & Vergari, S. (1996). Advocacy Coalitions, Policy Entrepreneurs, and Policy Change. *Policy Studies Journal, 24*(3), 420–434.

Roberts, N. C., & King, P. (1991). Policy Entrepreneurs: Their Activity Structure and Function in the Policy Process. *Journal of Public Administration Research and Theory, 1*(2), 147–175.

Saltman, R., Rico, A., & Boerma, W. (2005). *Primary Care in the Drivers Seat?* Maidenhead: Open University Press.

Steinmo, S., Thelen, K., & Longstreth, F. (1992). *Structuring Politics: Historical Institutionalism in Comparative Analysis*. Cambridge: Cambridge University Press.

# CHAPTER 6

# New Zealand: Context and the Performance Programme

**Abstract** In a dramatic contrast to the pay-for-performance scheme designed in England between 2001 and 2004, a much smaller scheme, the Performance Programme, was also being designed in New Zealand between the Ministry of Health and advisory groups of primary care stakeholders. Drawing on insights from 14 qualitative interviews with proximate policymakers, the context of and background to the policymaking are set out. The intentions of policymakers and the detailed story of the process to bring these to fruition are told in rich detail, often in the voices of the policymakers. The reader is allowed to see who was involved, what was done, how it was done and how it was implemented. Significant barriers that threatened the process and enablers that supported it are described and discussed.

**Keywords** Performance Programme • New Zealand's national health system • Pay-for-performance • Clinical autonomy

## BACKGROUND

In 1999, New Zealanders elected a majority coalition government led by the Labour Party after it had been nearly a decade out of office. Health services had high electoral salience during the election campaign. Laugesen (2000, p. 140) contends that health reformers had become "more attentive to voters' perceptions of reforms and the distribution of costs and

© The Author(s) 2018                                                  75
V. Smith, *Bargaining Power*,
https://doi.org/10.1007/978-981-10-7602-2_6

benefits" in New Zealand and that political revisions to reflect public opinion had begun to supplant technocratic blueprints for efficiency or health-care professional and provider interests in health policymaking.

Prior to its election victory, the Labour Party had set out a Manifesto dealing with health policy, "Labour on Health" (NZLP 1999), containing similar themes to those of the English Labour Party. In both countries, politicians were concerned about the gap between the expectations of taxpayers and health system performance. In New Zealand the concern was also to re-establish the "moral authority" of the national health system (NZLP 1999), whereas in England the Prime Minister sought to avoid a situation in which citizens "would begin to buy their way out and the NHS would spiral down to become a residualist safety net" (Stevens 2004).

In both countries a revolutionary programme of health reform had been introduced by the previous government, which had been largely imposed on an unwilling health sector (OECD 2004, p. 57). Each Labour Party distinguished itself from the previous administration by opposing key features of these reforms, replacing strategies based on competition and quasi-markets with greater cooperation, improved quality and a greater focus on prevention of chronic health conditions. As in England, the New Zealand Labour Party's core commitments were "to focus on patients not profits and to cut waiting times for surgery" (NZLP 1999, p. 2). But its objectives also addressed some different needs: for "restoration of a non-commercial system, with the focus on the provision of quality services"; "full involvement of the representatives of local communities in decisions about ... services in their region"; "significant improvements in the effectiveness of health services delivery to Māori and Pacific people" and a system in which "primary and secondary care will be well integrated." Health services had been allowed to become "run down, privatised and commercialized ... to the overwhelming alienation of the public" (NZLP 1999, p. 2). "Labour on Health" also signalled a focus on population-based and preventive health care, stating that the current system was "too focused on treatment services at the expense of improving the health of the community" and that the only accountability measures regularly reported on were financial rather than health service quality indicators. In future, it also stated, only "organisations which are funded by the state *and have a history of providing a quality service* will have funding arrangements which provide [this] security" (NZLP 1999, p. 4). Clinical accountability was to be given the same priority as financial accountability.

Quality and effectiveness were to be "the yardstick by which we measure the quality of the service" (NZLP 1999, p. 3).

"Labour on Health" sought to "raise the health status of New Zealanders and reduce the health status inequalities between different sections of the community" (NZLP 1999, pp. 3–4). The public health goals included reductions in smoking rates, incidence of asthma and diabetes, heart disease and high blood pressure, cancer-related mortality, poverty-related illnesses such as tuberculosis, meningitis, rickets and cellulitis and targets to increase immunisation rates (NZLP 1999, p. 5). Stating that "the key to improving the health status of New Zealanders in the long run hinges on public health and public policy measures more than on treatment" but that many of the illnesses "which are reducing life expectancy and requiring treatment are preventable within existing knowledge" (NZLP 1999, p. 10), the commitment was made to set and monitor national population health goals.

To restore the "moral authority" (NZLP 1999, p. 2) of the health system, democratic accountability mechanisms would be introduced together with the promise to restore affordable access to primary care so "that people's access to the health system is not restricted by their ability to pay" (NZLP 1999, p. 3). The plan to "return to a health system which allows people to have a say" (NZLP 1999, p. 2) would involve changes in governance and funding arrangements at the regional level and drawing primary care. The management of the interface between an integrated primary and secondary care sector would be "governed by organisations in which the community and consumers of services have a voice" (NZLP 1999, p. 4). At the national level, all functions for policy advice, funding, regulation and monitoring and public health services would be returned to the Ministry of Health and direct ministerial, and therefore parliamentary, control. Elected local representatives would form a majority on re-established District Health Boards, which would also be responsible for primary care. Decision-making would "once again be an open and publicly accountable process" (NZLP 1999). This was intended to improve the visibility of health services and, therefore, the accountability of health-care providers to citizens generally (Devlin 2001; Cumming 2002). It represented the re-introduction of a vertically integrated national health system, drawing all public health policy and funding back under the hierarchical control of the state.

Ensuring "that low cost quality primary health care services are available in areas of low income and high health need" (NZLP 1999, pp. 4,

13) and that "significant improvements will be made in the effectiveness of health service delivery to Māori and Pacific people" was also promised. The Manifesto promised "we will ensure that people's access to the health system is not restricted by their ability to pay" (NZLP 1999, p. 3).

New Zealand's semi-commercialised model of primary care delivery had become unaffordable for many New Zealanders. The primary care sector was already highly privatised in both production and consumption (Hay 1989) but the changes made in 1993 withdrew the subsidy for primary care entirely from most New Zealand adults (Flood 2001; Cumming 2011, p. 2). Research had shown that there were "significant and enduring health disparities relating to both ethnicity and deprivation" including a nine-year gap in life expectancy between Māori and non-Māori New Zealanders and between males living in the most deprived and least deprived geographical areas (Crampton 2000; Hefford 2005). The use of population-based funding formulae to determine funding levels for personal health services so that funding could be redistributed based on need, with targets for delivery of preventive as well as curative services, and the introduction of the requirement for people to enrol on registers for health care were all foreshadowed.

Major changes to funding arrangements for primary care (NZLP 1999, p. 12) were also signalled. The Labour Party also proposed to prevent public funding being spent on contracts with for-profit organisations. This signalled a major challenge to the network of existing Independent Practitioners' Associations (IPAs) which had formed in the 1990s to facilitate contracting between general practitioners and regional funders. These were primarily doctor-owned private companies (Gauld 2006) and most had adopted contracts for referred services budget management offered by regional funders during this period. These contracts had the intention "to curb growth in referred services expenditure … and typically rewarded reduced expenditure by allowing organisations to keep a proportion of the savings for agreed projects" (Referred Services Advisory Group 2002, p. 16). They had delivered savings which funded significant new health service developments by IPAs (Crampton 2004) and those other general practice consortia (including some community organisations in rural communities), which adopted them and funded clinical governance initiatives for their members. There were 30 IPAs in 1999, representing over 75 per cent of general practitioners (Malcolm 1999a), and "almost all" had taken on responsibility for budgets for pharmaceutical services with some also having budgets for laboratory services. The level of savings obtained by some large IPAs and the ability for these Associations to determine how to use these savings without consultation with the community was specifically criticised in the Labour Party Manifesto. A participant in this research suggests that "there was a perception that the budget-holding exercises of the previous … years had resulted in inappropriate and inequitable capture of funding … and IPAs … gained a lot."

Primary care organisations formed within the network of community-governed not-for-profit health centres typically did not take up budget-management contracts. Evaluation in 1999 indicated that IPAs, who benefited most from these contracts, were those with high historical levels of expenditure on referred services and high utilisation rates serving "well-off populations with general practitioner availability well above the national average" (Malcolm 2004). This concern was shared by both Labour and National politicians: another participant commented that "their organisations have ended up with enormous amounts of money sitting in a bank and even [a spokesperson within the National Party] just goes apoplectic, it is $80 million because it is not spent on health … and it was utterly up to the Trust [of the IPA] how they decided to spend it."

The Manifesto announced that any contracting for services with primary care organisations by the new District Health Boards would be with non-profit groups with adequate community or consumer representation.

A path needed to be trodden carefully between a variety of heterogeneous general practice and primary health-care groups and interests, including the network of IPAs which had established clinical governance processes for their member practices during the 1990s, and the new network of other consortia of general practice organisations and Māori and Pacific organisations which had developed to deliver services to their people during the same period.

In New Zealand clinical quality assurance had largely developed through regional professionally led initiatives arising in the IPAs and other similar primary health management organisations that had developed clinical governance approaches to improve the quality and resource management of pharmaceutical prescribing and laboratory test referrals among their members (Barnett 2004). Researchers noted that evidence of "substantial inter-practitioner variation in patterns of primary care activity has been established for over a decade" and that the literature tended to explain this by practice and practitioner attributes including professional uncertainty and supplier-induced demand. This study found considerable variability in medical practice after controlling for case-mix and patient and practitioner attributes and concluded that some 10 per cent of this variation was attributable to physician attributes (Davis 2002). Complementing general practitioner-led peer group networks, the IPAs and similar organisations implemented "comprehensive information systems, computerised practice registers ... personalised feedback on prescribing behaviour and laboratory use and peer group discussion of guidelines" (Malcolm 1999a, p. 1341) to address this picture of considerable variation in practice, which was largely based on volume rather than price (in which prescribing members prescribe many more drugs but not necessarily more expensive drugs than low-cost prescribers). Savings varied between levels of 5–10 per cent of referred services budgets (Malcolm 1999b).

Associated with these developments in organised clinical governance had been supportive national initiatives (Barnett 2004), including a national programme of capacity-building for quality, including clinical guidelines development, in the 1990s and the formation of organisations such as the New Zealand Guidelines Group in 1996 and the Clinical Leaders Association of New Zealand in 1998.

Key elements of the "Labour on Health" proposals were a challenge to the aspirations of organisations representing most general practitioners. By contrast, community-governed not-for-profit primary care practices employed 3 per cent of practitioners but these worked in multi-disciplinary teams with other health professionals. In comparison with for-profit practices, they served a younger, poorer, largely non-European population, with higher levels of certain types of health issues, including asthma, diabetes and skin infections (Crampton 2004). They and their representative organisations had "long taken a broader population perspective beyond the traditional general practice focus" (Smith 2007, p. 17). Whereas the focus of the IPAs was on engagement with their general practitioner members, the focus of non-profit practices was strongly on engagement with their local community. The values and perspectives of these practices and organisations were better aligned with the proposed changes outlined in the "Labour on Health" document. In some regions, these practices joined meso-organisations which were not IPAs but offered similar services to them.

The proposed changes were also in sharp contrast with the health reforms of 1993 which had been a top-down, rationalist and technically driven approach, and non-consultative in its process of design and decision-making (Finlayson 2000). Davis and other commentators (Tuohy 1999) also note the subsequent unravelling of much of this policy intent during the process of implementation, as both medical and public opposition to the changes grew during this phase. In Finlayson's assessment, "funders' ability to counteract the power of the medical profession was impeded by their lack of information and expertise necessary for the negotiation with doctors." She concludes that key aspects of the 1993 reforms proved impossible to introduce successfully because much of the policy was based on inadequate assumptions about its environment and because implementation was not a "neutral non-political stage of the policymaking process ... rather the whole process has the potential to be highly politicised, especially when key groups have not been involved in the formulation of policy" (Finlayson 2000). It was in the context of this pre-history that the incoming Labour government embarked upon its counter-revolutionary changes in health policy in 1999 (Starke 2010).

## A Ministerial/Civil Service Partnership

Once elected in late 1999, the incoming Labour government began to implement its Manifesto commitments immediately to ensure results could be delivered within its three-year term of office. The new Minister of Health, Hon. Annette King (hereafter "the Minister"), and the Director-General of Health met promptly after ministerial appointments were made. These two entered into a strong partnership to implement the reform programme. A participant observed that working with the new Minister,

> it was a very Westminster "here is what we want to do, can you tell us how we would do it?" ... It was what you would expect and it was very very constructive. [The Ministry] would do the work, test it with her, if it needed to go to Cabinet and come back, very supportive, very willing to be driving but to be patient; ... it was a good partnership, each ... doing [their] own roles which meant that we could get some difficult stuff done.

Although researchers in the New Zealand Treasury offered the new government advice to establish a new set of relationships with primary care providers, especially general practitioners, and noted that "there were few incentives on primary care providers to consider the wider implications of their decisions for the rest of the sector and [that] the delivery of primary care is imperfectly coordinated with other services" (Mays 2000), the advice was not heeded.

## THE GOVERNMENT STRATEGIES

The development of two major health strategies, the New Zealand Health Strategy, published in December 2000, and the Primary Health Care Strategy (PHCS), published in February 2001, was undertaken with widespread clinical and community input (King 2001) on each strategy. The New Zealand Health Strategy has as its predominant theme the need to reduce inequalities in health care (King 2000). Governance changes, structural changes in financing arrangements, goals to improve performance on particular conditions and an injection of new money were the chosen mechanisms to achieve this. The Strategy established 13 population health objectives to reduce the impact of disease and poor lifestyle choices.

The PHCS which followed, therefore, set out,

> a new direction for primary health care with a greater emphasis on population health and the role of the community, health promotion and preventive care, the need to involve a range of professionals and the advantages of funding based on population needs rather than fees-for-service. (King 2001)

Treasury advice to establish new relationships with primary care providers, especially general practitioners, was noted but not heeded.

The development of the two strategies was seen by some participants in this research as part of a continuing struggle between general practitioners and the Labour Party over primary care health policy (which occurred most intensely over issues associated with private billing by practitioners). The stresses in this relationship were still fresh in the minds of several research participants even though these events had occurred over ten years before the development of new primary health-care policies. On balance, while they are a contextual factor which deterred whole-hearted engagement of some sections of the general practice interest groups representing most general practitioners, they are incidental to the rationale for the PHCS.

The Minister personally led the development of the New Zealand Health Strategy and the PHCS. She confirms that the Prime Minister left it all to her as Minister of Health and that there was a "bit of a myth about [the Prime Minister] and Health ... but she wasn't [in the role of Minister of Health in the previous Labour government] very long ... and [Labour] had a very detailed manifesto in Health." The Ministry of Health did the detailed work in developing the published strategy. The Minister says that "the strategy was actually written by the Ministry with my input and the input of people ... who were very aware of how it works [such as] having been a doctor up the East Coast."

The heterogeneous general practice community in New Zealand had various responses to the proposed changes, according to a leader of a major IPA. Clinicians were excited the importance of primary care was recognised, but had their strongest focus on patients who walked in the door, feeling a high level of commitment to advocacy for them. They did not understand "disparity" in access to health services well. They felt little responsibility for a population-based approach to health. There was a pervasive feeling that they were paid for seeing patients in consultation, not for those outside the practice register or who chose not to visit the practice (O'Malley 2003), and they did not like the targeting of health care to a particular group of patients. They felt that all who were ill needed the same level of clinical response. General practitioners did not feel that they had the expertise to develop health promotion or health education strategies or to use population health tools as required by the new PHCS. Participants interviewed for this research saw the PHCS as having many laudable elements but containing a fundamental threat to doctors by what they saw as explicit proposals to augment clinical leadership and clinical governance of their practice with a primary care team-based and community-governed approach. One participant says,

> there were lots of things that made general practitioners very tense. General practitioners associated Labour with being anti-general practitioner. [They] are actually a private business and if you don't build that into your policy you will strike resistance and fail in certain ways.

As another participant put it, "It was a turbulent time. Government and the [primary care] groups were in a major conflict around how government funding was rolled out.... [The Prime Minister] had had a low view of GPs."

This period of policymaking was described by a participant as engendering

> a major cultural shift ... [in which] what had held them together through the 90s and supported a lot of the innovation they got into such as cell

groups, utilization review and feedback, performance improvement activities ... were abandoned as inappropriate in the new environment ...

Unlike the spontaneous emergence of organisational and governance forms in primary care during the 1990s, changes were quickly imposed by the Ministry of Health and District Health Boards (DHBs), despite misgivings in parts of the primary health-care sector. The opportunity for organisations to re-form as intermediate non-profit organisations, PHOs, to be funded on a capitated needs-based formula, was set out. Clear criteria were set down for an organisation to become a PHO. Research has established that "a hierarchical mode of governance was in fact implemented quickly, with mechanisms to ensure political accountability to the government" (Barnett 2009, p. 118) through the new District Health Boards. New rules specified that services delivered with public funding must be directed towards improving and maintaining the health of the population as well as first-line services to treat the unwell; involve the communities in their governing processes and show that they are responsive to communities' priorities and needs; demonstrate that all their providers and practitioners can influence the organisation's decision-making rather than one group being dominant; and be not-for-profit organisations fully and openly accountable for all public funds they receive. PHOs were required to identify initiatives to improve the health of their enrolled population and work with groups who have poor health or were missing out on services to address their needs. This set of requirements was incompatible with the ownership and governance arrangements of most existing IPAs and would require them to radically change their mode of operation to comply with the requirements and access the new funding for primary care services. While a general practice could voluntarily become a member of a PHO, there were considerable financial incentives to do so once new funding for primary care was announced. Only through PHOs could new levels of subsidy be gained. By 2005 77 PHOs covering 3.9 million New Zealanders'had enrolled for their services.

## WHO WAS INVOLVED

Pay-for-performance was not mentioned in the New Zealand Health Strategy and the PHCS, though the Health Strategy spoke of setting standards and performance targets and rewarding achievement of these. The introduction and approval of the pay-for-performance policy proposal came through a working group, led by a senior civil servant, which had been set up to find ways to manage pharmaceutical prescribing and referrals to services more equitably within a population-based funding framework, now that budget-management contracts were no longer available. Resembling the technically driven and rationalist policymaking process developed during the 1990s (Finlayson 2000), it was nevertheless more inclusive, readily adopting ideas from the primary health-care sector, than the process which was used to develop the health policy proposals implemented in 1993. It is described by a participant:

> The idea ... that it would be very good to incentivise certain performance measures ... grew out of the nexus of communication between the Ministry and the sector ... the primary health care sector itself had measures and some of the groupings of general practices had gone quite a long way down the pathway.... [The Ministry] were wanting to shift the focus from the one-to-one walk in the door, fix the big toe, to "you have an enrolled population, we want you keeping them healthy, we want measures that are collective and for the PHO to be able to influence."

The Ministry of Health wished to build on what existed, such as the utilisation review and clinical governance systems which IPAs had developed. This participant says that officials were keen to say "look [they] had this in place prior, could [they] not use something like this in future, could it not be national." Understanding that it was "fertile ground—[the sector] had done some of the work" and that "[it was possible] to use some of their ideas, [not] rubbishing the structures that were there, [but to] use them to build into the future" assisted in the building of acceptance of the changes. A participant in the design team confirms:

> Key elements such as utilisation review and feedback, comparison of individual utilisation patterns versus that of a wider group [was] what we were trying to preserve. In essence that was the nucleus of the 90s that we were trying to take forward into the next stage, but shifting the focus from "pharms" and "labs" into a population health environment compatible with the PHO model and scalable and reproducible across the whole country.

Another participant acknowledges that "the government were trying to say, 'You guys had done some performance stuff and we are keen to try to understand that and put it into this new paradigm—I credit them for that.'"

A Referred Services Advisory Group (RSAG) was convened by a senior Ministry of Health official in 2001 to provide advice on suitable ways of funding referred services, how to develop and support clinical governance, suitable performance measures and information needs and other tools (Referred Services Advisory Group 2002). A participant explains one motive:

> We needed to move away from rewarding savings on historical budgets and instead reward quality and at the same time put much more focus on equity. Under the existing arrangements, the more disadvantaged populations tended to have low levels of "pharms" and "labs" spending and were missing out—on drugs and lab tests as well as on the opportunity to benefit from the savings achieved by [other] general practitioners.

The RSAG was tasked to advise the Ministry, among other things, on "appropriate incentives for organisations to manage referred services within a predetermined budget" (Referred Services Advisory Group 2002, p. 4). The RSAG Report's subtitle demonstrates the dominance of concerns about equity, "Building towards equity, quality and better health outcomes." Heavily dominated by academic and funder interests, it met on six occasions between October 2001 and August 2002. The report's recommendations cover the general approach for funding pharmaceuticals and laboratory tests and provide an exemplary set of indicators, a payment and information management framework and a clinical governance framework together with an implementation plan. The new approach recommended "financial rewards for quality practice, as opposed to financially reward under-spending of a budget based on historic spending levels" (Referred Services Advisory Group 2002, p. 7). To do so, the report stated that a set of nationally consistent quality indicators needed to be developed and that strategies by IPAs in developing among general practitioners a "sense of collegiality and accountability, greater sensitivity to quality issues, acceptance of the need for evidence-based decision making, exposure to peer review and building a sense of identity within a new and broadly based organisational framework" could be built on (Referred Services Advisory Group 2002). An exemplary set of 29 indicators was set out in the Report, drawing on the work done for a primary care organisation, First Health Ltd., which had been published in the *New Zealand Medical Journal* in 2002 (Gribben 2002). Only some of these relate to referred services. The set contains proposed indicators such as advice to smokers, childhood and older person flu immunizations, blood pressure screening, action plans for asthmatics and diabetes management processes. These resemble the breadth and potential for impact on health outcomes of the QOF in England and are consistent with the most pressing health problems noted in the New Zealand Health Strategy. It is in fact a blueprint for incentivising quality and for improving health outcomes generally. The report notes that the commitment by government to a substantial increase in funding for primary care services justified an increased expectation by funders on improved quality of service. The report goes on to emphasise the importance of an improved and nationally consistent information database to enable assessment of compliance with quality practice and of the availability of clinical governance systems to support practices in improving quality and proposed a funding model which offers up to 2 per cent of annual average per capita spending, including on referred services, as a reward for PHOs achieving the maximum quality score.

The next step was to establish a group of providers, professional groups and funders to oversee a consultative, Internet-based process for developing a broad set of quality indicators for PHOs, with performance measures and targets. The full participation of medical practitioners in the decision-making around selection of quality indicators was seen to be essential. A participant recalls that people "had their own measures in place and they were very attached to them. The general feeling was that indicators were an important tool but that each group of GPs should be able to determine their own set."

First, after a debate to decide on indicators, an Internet-based Delphi process was implemented. A participant recalls that,

> thirty general practitioners were in the sample who suggested indicators, they did not have to meet but we did a lot of analysis between cycles and if someone wanted to get rid of some indicator the reason was provided and little graphs were sent out; ... we looked at the attrition rate as people had to ... score it and we used lots of different ways [to monitor and encourage engagement].... The only resistance we had was from people who wanted a more rigorous process.

However, participation levels dropped. Others suggest the process became undermined by technical problems and absenteeism and that small numbers of participants stayed the course of the process. Following this process, in September 2003 a Clinical Performance Indicator Advisory Group was established to provide advice on implementation of a set of clinical indicators and had commissioned Otago University's Wellington School of Medicine and Health Sciences to develop an indicator assessment tool and report with recommendations for the process for identifying and deciding upon indicators.

The second step was to form another project which was handed to joint Chairs representing DHBs and the Ministry respectively. Their task was to consider management of referred services within an incentivised framework. The Referred Services Expert Advisory Group (RSEAG) engaged a large group of stakeholders to come together to debate and design a pay-for-performance programme for primary care. By contrast with the rationalist and technocratic approach taken in the design phase of this policymaking process, the implementation phase was intended to obtain maximum engagement with key funder and provider stakeholders. The Joint Chairs of the RSEAG themselves were carefully chosen. One was a general practitioner and ex-general manager of a primary care network organisation who had been appointed to a senior advisory role in the Ministry of Health to support the implementation of the PHCS. Another was employed in a large DHB, who had also had considerable experience in managing budget-holding and budget-management contracts during the 1990s. He knew the sector leaders very well and his management experience complemented the clinical experience of the other co-Chair. In fact they had worked together during the 1990s and were instrumental in developing a capitated funding approach for general practice that was widely accepted by providers in their region. In this, these two policymakers resembled leaders of the English initiative— outsiders to the core civil service who could be considered to have high experience and credibility built in the earlier era of market-oriented funder/profession relationships. These skills and relationships were seen as necessary and useful if they could be carried into the new collaborative, community-oriented era.

When it came to the selection of members for the RSEAG and the design process itself, the Chairs had a clear strategy. As a participant recalls:

Basically [they] got everybody inside the tent ... chose the stakeholders, the people to get into the tent and they were of course all the troublemakers, all the people with very strong opinions on it; plus ... moderated that a bit by making sure ... [there was] vocal Māori and Pacific presence there.

Members were primarily chosen for their expertise. They included general practitioners, pathologists, pharmacists, people with an inequalities perspective. Another recalls:

> People selected were identified on the basis of expertise and experience with actually making something happen in relation to clinical governance, not on the basis of representation of professional groups. That particular approach caused tensions. The reality was most of the people were also members of national groups but [they were chosen] ... because they were recognized as leaders in this area.

Within the different interests, a distinction could be made between those with experience of organised general practice—the IPAs—and those general practitioners who were focused on high needs and equity of provision. A participant from within the first group comments:

> [T]he membership reflected the ideology of the times—quite sensibly the government were trying to say [the sector] have [sic] done some performance stuff and we are keen to try to understand that and put it into this new paradigm—I credit them for that thinking but the ideology was more important ... it was a state-directed programme.

Some practitioner members of the group were reported by participants as later disowning the resulting programme. A participant acknowledges "At the end of it would I say the College [of General Practice] had a sense of ownership around the programme?—absolutely not for reasons which are quite complex ... it is a question of control."

The RSEAG met over a nine-month period. There was vigorous debate among members about how existing systems and resources for clinical leadership would be affected. Considerable anxiety was voiced among IPA leaders that their systems and resources for clinical leadership would be imperilled in this environment and income streams upon which they had come to rely would be closed off. A participant explains:

> Performance improvement activities had been funded through pharmaceutical, and in some cases laboratory, budget-holding ... which allowed them to undertake all these activities that had mobilized general practice and led to a lot of the performance improvement initiatives.... These people had been the leaders in the 1990s and had personally led a whole round of innovation and entrepreneurial drive and that needed a home.

The need to address health inequalities was vigorously championed by members with experience of community-based primary care service delivery in regions with high health needs and by Māori and Pacific members. The perceived need to remove the wide variation in referred services expenditure was not explained by patient factors and pointed instead to inequity of utilisation. A participant says:

> [They] needed to have some transparency around equity in budget setting.... Take [an IPA with] some of the highest pharmaceutical utilisation in the country—how would you set a "pharms" budget ... using a national formula? They would never have any savings; ... [the IPA] had got to get expenditure down to the national norm.

An equity focus rather than cost control was important because the international experience with pay-for-performance is that schemes can aggravate inequalities in the short term. The problem of cost containment had largely been tackled already:

> The driver of pharmaceutical budget holding had been growth in pharmaceutical expenditure, but actually Pharmac (New Zealand's central purchaser of pharmaceuticals) had that under control, so why bother? In respect of labs that was the start of the period [when] labs were themselves ... moved off fee-for-service and onto fixed contracts meaning they were carrying the volume and price risk.

This meant that quality improvement had to be the rationale for the project, requiring a fundamental shift in focus. The participant further explains, "At the end of the day [it] was about improving performance in primary health care." There was also an acceptance that "all patients are in PHOs, all practices are in PHOs, this has got to be a model which is available for all, not just negotiated idiosyncratically IPA by IPA."

This in turn raised concerns. Another participant says, "There are some organisations who feel uneasy about funders wanting to get into performance and quality improvement because it is seen as an area where professional control is fundamental." There was sympathy for those concerns.

> [It was necessary] to understand why people would be concerned ... "do I want to get into bed with government, how could I protect myself?" ... Mostly they wanted to do well for their patients.... [They] had to walk in the shoes [of those organisations]—it is classic change management really.

## HOW IT WAS DONE

As one participant describes it, it was like herding cats, to come up with indicators that were appropriate, with clinical and financial indicators and a focus on Pacific people, Māori and people with high needs all in place. There were often 20 people in the meetings. One of the Chairs was reported by participants to play a key role in getting the dynamics of the group working well and ensuring the process was based on consensus (private conversation). Another believed the vigour of well-managed debate created a more robust policy framework.

> Do you want everybody thinking the same and it being easy or do you want a bunch of people who think differently.... But at the end of the day you get a better product ... because you have ironed out all the "ifs" and the "buts".

The RSEAG included Māori and Pacific members who advocated strongly for the needs of their communities. A participant recalls,

> Areas of real dispute included whether or not to make recording ethnicity a condition of entry to the programme; some were won and some didn't get through. Some got manipulated and changed, so they became ineffective in changing behaviour.

Another area of dispute was whether to focus on one or two major targets with large health impacts such as smoking: "Which is the biggest preventable cause of death in New Zealand. Why didn't we choose that first?"

The issue of incentivising performance was not prominent in the debates. One participant recalls, "I am not sure the government was actually trying to implement pay-for-performance." Another confirms that the use of financial incentives was to strengthen the role of PHOs and bring in the general practitioners and nurses for education. Participants felt that the financial incentives were used because of evidence that they worked but their primary purpose was not to incentivise practitioners.

This differentiates the New Zealand scheme fundamentally from the English one. In England the locus of impact of the incentives was to be the health actions taken by the individual general practitioner with patients on their register. The locus of impact of the New Zealand scheme was on the actions of PHOs to encourage providers of primary care services in their community to focus on preventive health care. The incentives and processes associated with this scheme operated at the level of PHO policy-making and practice, at an arm's-length from the health actions of practitioners or from the clinical governance systems which supported quality improvement in general practice. The same incentives for individual general practitioners to engage with policymaking which, it has been seen, animated the negotiations in England were not present to the same extent in the New Zealand policymaking process.

A strong principle was agreed by all parties in New Zealand that the money went to the PHOs rather than automatically into practice income as it would do in the scheme in England. There was no antecedent policy of incentivising general practitioners directly as there was in England. Even IPAs' budget-management savings had to be re-invested in clinical governance systems and health services. The survey conducted in 1998 had reported that IPAs considered "the retention of savings for personal benefits as both unprofessional and unethical" (Malcolm 2000).

The risk of crowding out other valued behaviours was also a concern to the group, explained by a participant as follows:

> It is small by comparison with QOF because the committee didn't want people to spend all their clinical hours focusing on these indicators some of which might not be relevant. It's a burden for practices to do all this extra activity so why would we get them to do activity which would not necessarily improve health? … So [they] were reluctant to add in more.

The discussions were seen as convivial—one participant commented that "there were no stand up rows and walking out" and another felt:

> The dynamics in the group were great; … we had about the right amount of people with the right types of views and common agreement that we would debate the hell out of them.

However, some members with experience of organised general practice contributed to a pattern of disengagement from active participation in the debates, both during the process of implementation design and later when the Performance Programme (PP) was launched.

Sometimes the technical challenges of the task were sufficient to transcend deep-seated differences in interests and priorities. Officials were sometimes surprised at the way members of the group appeared to place the interests of their organisations second to the technical requirements of designing an effective scheme. A participant said:

I did a presentation to … the Ministry—it's another one of those vivid memories where you go to the Ministry and say this is where it is going and its completely wrong and [the official] looked at me and said why on earth would YOU tell me this—if we correct the formula it will get worse for [your PHO]; … this attitude about PHO motives persists today.

Another says:

There was intense distrust between the Ministry and general practice—always has been and always will be. They have different goals. The Ministry of Health is a bureaucracy and wants to maintain itself and serve its political masters. General practice is not that animal—it has its own role and different parts have different goals like ensuring the financial viability of doctors or maintaining their power and dominance and access to the money and other socialist parts of general practice see the role to improve the health of the population. General practice in New Zealand didn't want to see the closeness of the relationship with the government that exists in the UK.

The plurality of general practice forms was reflected in these debates. The views of the members associated with IPA contrasted with those from other types of primary health management organisations and non-profit groups with largely salaried staff operating as primary care health centres in areas of high socio-economic need. One participant said that "this is what [they were] trying to achieve out of PHOs … almost a reaction against the IPA-type model…. The population focus, community-linked, focus on inequalities was in the strategy, not focusing on making a dollar."

In the design stage, the Chairs worked hard to achieve policy recommendations based on group consensus, rather than unanimity. No attempt was made to achieve formal approval from representative primary health-care provider organisations or the general practice leadership in New Zealand, about the recommendations for the scheme. Members of the group were not mandated, nor expected, to speak on behalf of their organisations. As has been reported above, some, subsequent to the approval of the framework by ministers, later disowned elements of it.

The final set of 13 indicators reflected compromise, pressure of time, ready availability of data and a belief that it was better to "build the infrastructure and expectations around measuring something" which could then evolve.

The group utilised the assistance of the University of Otago Wellington School of Medicine and Health Sciences to complete the selection of a small set of 13 indicators for the first phase of implementation. The selected indicators had to be the subject of existing data-collection processes so did not always directly correlate with improved health status. This issue of data availability also reflected past disputes between IPAs, which had been seen as reluctant to share information, and other community-governed organisations which were keen to collaborate and share information and strategies to improve services with one another. A participant believes,

> One of the principles of the [doctors in the 1990s] regime was "we own the data". When you strip away the rhetoric you get "if we own the data we own the system. You can buy it but we will tell you which bits you can buy." ... [T]his really illuminates the whole system of PHOs versus IPAs. IPAs own the data but PHOs can say we are the community and it is our data—why shouldn't we share it?

Another group member recalls that some general practitioners were very concerned about privacy risks and that data relating to some indicators such as mental health conditions and breast screening could become identifiable (personal communication).

The set of indicators which were finally selected for the launch of the PP were of three types: clinical; process indicators (focusing on the ability of the PHO to support population health and quality interventions); and financial indicators of pharmaceutical and laboratory expenditure against benchmarks of indicative budgets weighted for unmet need. The clinical indicators were those which could be drawn from national databases in a pragmatic step to enable the programme to get under way. It was decided that implementation of a second set of provisional indicators would need to be contingent on more work at the practice and PHO level. These were to be focused on chronic disease (including smoking status, statins use, recording of chronic disease and certain data relating to cardiovascular risk, diabetes, urinary tract infection investigation and tests for iron deficiency).

The clinical indicators constituted 60 per cent of the total possible score, financial indicators 30 per cent and 10 per cent for process achievements. A double weighting for achievement for high-needs populations which could be identified within a PHO total enrolled population was provisioned. The rewards could be used for extending or introducing health programmes, quality initiatives, continuous quality improvement infrastructure, rewarding practices for effort or funding professional development, as agreed between the PHO and the DHB.

A final report to the Minister of Health, detailing the "emergent approach" with a "good level of sector buy-in," was completed in May 2005 (Ministry of Health 2005, p. 16) with recommendations for the implementation of the programme. In all, the process took a further two years from the completion of the 2002 RSAG report to complete the detailed policy design for decision. Together with the subsequent implementation projects, the whole design process took five years to complete prior to PP commencement and a further two years for implementation.

## IMPLEMENTATION

Feedback on the draft framework for the PP had been sought, as in England, from the primary care sector in a national road show in 2004. The set of indicators and the funding framework were approved in July 2005. Twenty-nine PHOs participated in the first phase of roll-out (a number higher than expected), rising to 42 the following year. The number of participants in 2007 rose to 81 of the then 82 PHOs. Achievement levels against the indicators averaged 81 per cent in 2009. Payments were made six-monthly to the PHO, based upon performance reported to them in two previous quarterly progress reports. For a PHO with 70,000 enrolled patients and average achievement (81 per cent), the annual performance payment would be just over $330,000. This might have resulted in an annual payment of over $20,000 per practice (based on an average enrolled population of 5000 per practice).

This was in fact a significant amount of money. However, the size of the potential rewards for practices was not promoted by the Ministry and was a surprise to participants in the governance group of the PP after its roll-out; nor was it promoted after roll-out. Doctors' representatives may well have been misled by this. They were surprised by how much funding was available but not being accessed when they discovered the amounts budgeted for the programme.

Some years later when the governance group for the PP had been extended and included more members from large general practice organisations, a discussion was held about the funding available for the PP. A participant on the group recalls that it was said, there was a line item for $35 million but they didn't expect to spend it because people wouldn't achieve the targets. In the room GPs suddenly had a quick discussion and said so if we lowered the targets we could get all that money and the Ministry people nearly fell off their chairs. It was a good example of the thinking of different groups.

## BARRIERS AND ENABLERS OF THE POLICYMAKING PROCESS

### *Redistribution of General Practice Resources*

As in England, the pay-for-performance programme was a part of a larger primary health-care strategy. New Zealand's Labour politicians in 1999 sought to implement a "counter-revolution" to restore universality, hierarchical governance and community engagement in health services (Starke 2010) and resolve inequity of access to primary care services. The PHCS in New Zealand moved the funding from a targeted, fee-for-service arrangement to a universal, capitated environment for general practice, with higher funding levels to reduce co-payments to patients, and to support these mechanisms, particularly the introduction of capitation, the state also needed to achieve the enrolment of all citizens with a PHO. The requirement to allocate a unique National Health Index identifier to all patients accompanied this initiative and provided a system for tracking service use and a population denominator for measuring practice and primary health organisation performance.

In practice this meant that PHOs and their general practices had to be supported to utilise data about their enrolled population and plan resource utilisation in a capitated funding environment. One participant confirms "we were trying to make sure that at a PHO level there was accountability for an enrolled population ... keeping them healthy, we want measures that are collective and for the PHO to be able to influence ... members/ practices."

In a second strategy to redistribute general practice resources, additional funding in the form of higher subsidies for visits to practices was made available to regions with high socio-economic deprivation. Availability of these higher subsidies was contingent on practices agreeing to limit co-payments to patients. Until it was resolved, by reinstating an earlier fee oversight regime, the roll-out of the new higher levels of subsidy for communities with high socio-economic deprivation was thought to be at risk of stalling.

An area of health inequality which particularly concerned the Labour government (NZLP 1999) was the need for "significant improvement … in the effectiveness of health service delivery to Māori and Pacific peoples." At all stages of the design and implementation process of this policymaking episode, the voices, needs and concerns of Māori and Pacific communities were strongly reflected. This was a primary purpose of the PP's counter-balancing initiatives to deter under-servicing. Population-based treatment and screening initiatives were not core business for general practice and took both time and resources that practices did not believe they had. One participant thought,

> You need to target to improve access. For [some] areas … which needed to reduce their utilisation down to a national norm, within that they needed to increase utilization for some. It required a level of sophistication that was very, very challenging and that is why it was absolutely critical to have the [Māori and Pacific voices] in the room as advocates for those populations, and the need for clinical leaders to step up to make a difference to health inequalities…. [The Māori and Pacific members] were very powerful in that group. They weren't put off by the need to be outspoken.

Another participant recalls that

> the old style fund-holding worked well in some areas but where it didn't work well was [in] inequalities and this was really in vogue back then. It was part of "the new". Closing the Gaps [in outcomes between European New Zealanders and Māori New Zealanders] was one of the really significant things Labour came out with when it was releasing the strategy so … designing a Referred Services stream that didn't rely on historic budgets (because that is what promoted the inequality) meant that it drove it down an incentives programme route.

For some it did not go far enough or fast enough. A participant confirms,

> Areas of real dispute included whether or not to make ethnicity a condition of entry to the programme, some were won, some didn't get through…. The other thing we kept saying was why should we pay for achievement for the dominant population when there is no problem. Why wouldn't we … only pay for results for the priority population—which might shift depending on the indicator … we didn't win that debate.

One participant subsequently reflected:

One thing I feel really positive about is the focus on inequalities across the programme. While that was a principle at the front end at the start of the process there was no detail about how that was going to be achieved. In particular, it was the participation of [a particular member of the group].

## *Balancing Funder Interests and Clinical Autonomy*

Participants describe a conflict between funder interests and clinical autonomy in three major ways during the policymaking process for both the larger PHCS and the PP design: seeking to influence health actions of general practitioners, the principle of clinically led quality improvement and fee levels. The first two are focused on here.

While it was understood that it was "the natural desire of independent businesses to be independent of government … if government is putting more money in then there has to be a balance between government being specific about what they are going to get for that money." It was believed that doctors had firm views about things like the patient relationship. But there was uneasiness among doctors "about funders wanting to get into performance and quality improvement…. This area is one of the defining characteristics of a profession." Much discussion focused on "the boundary between professional issues and funder issues." Another on the group confirmed that "the old debate between PHOs and IPAs about who has real control—the community board of governance or the health professionals … was another arm wrestle going on…. General practice in New Zealand didn't want to see the closeness of the relationship with the government that exists in the UK. Go back to the Bassett era [a former Labour Minister of Health] and the attempt to control general practice and … they saw it as a victory over the forces of darkness.".

A fundamental division occurred over whether the process of designing a quality improvement system should be clinically led (primarily by general practitioners) or driven by community priorities. A participant, in commenting on who was involved in design of the policy, confirmed that,

it was a big call to have a multi-disciplinary group; part of the issue was that … what you wanted delivered wasn't delivered by general practitioners anyway…. There is more to primary health than general practitioners and they didn't like you saying that but it was true…. If we go back to totally doctor-dominated general practice then we have lost all the idea that the PHOs weren't just about going to the doctor.

The comment implicitly recognised that the product of the policy implementation process was not specifically directed at general practitioners but at the wider primary health-care professional team.

Many participants were not concerned about the make-up of the group or the role for a broad range of primary care professionals in setting clinical standards, as it was consistent with the way community-governed, not-for-profit practices operated. For IPA-oriented members this was a more-fundamental issue of control of a core aspect of professional identity—independence.

There were big debates about who should be at the table. For one participant the issue was simple:

> This was a state-directed programme. I have often reflected that I don't think a single thing [some participants] said ... was reflected in the programme that was rolled out ... [such as] peer-led, based on feedback and performance data to individuals, the data referenced to colleagues and the group as a whole and using clinical meetings based on the evidence and outlier management visit ... a non-judgmental, peer accountability process.

Among some representatives of general practice it was believed that the intent of the PHCS was to replace clinical leadership and governance with community leadership and governance, and an attempt to make "the union/community-owned model of healthcare ... the New Zealand health care system model." By contrast with processes in New Zealand, one participant describes how in England "the Secretary of State [for Health] was on stage talking and he was entirely comfortable with talking about a GP-led system."

### Shaping Patterns of Interaction Between the State and Interest Groups

A history of adversarial relationships between some parts of the general practice sector and the Labour Party had always increased the difficulties faced by Labour governments to build positive working relationships with all parts of the general practice profession. Health Minister King commented that "I think it goes right back to the first Labour government when they wanted to have socialised medicine.... [A]nd general practice was an important part of it ... and the fight started back then." She noted that by contrast with politicians in England who had "quite a lot of support at times from the BMA ... that was very rare [for a New Zealand politician to] ever get a compliment." Another dates the lack of trust of some professional leaders of general practice to "the 1940s since the first attempt to get the Social Welfare Act together post-war ... but they walked away from it and said no we don't want to be a part of it and the subsidies that were there got smaller and smaller and the rest is history." Another spoke of "the stories that rolled around Labour conferences—bad doctors hadn't fallen in with the social security legislation in 1938" and went on to say, "Actually I don't think it served anybody particularly well: we can't change history."

Like the English policymakers, much effort in New Zealand was directed at demonstrating a new collaborative approach and seeking win/win solutions to policy dilemmas, but through consultation with stakeholders in primary health care, not negotiation with appointed representatives of general practice. Speaking generally about the whole primary health-care changes, King said, "I knew I had to bring [the general practitioners] along because it wasn't only about what they charged, but getting them to think differently about a health team; ... with health it was a relationship issue ... it really was about relationships, first, second and third, and money ... I used force of personality, partly." "[If you] looked at what had happened to [previous Labour ministers] ... in the end they would fight ... and they would undermine you ... so I had to do it by power of persuasion."

She also believed:

> They wanted the money because primary health care was struggling in comparison to someone who was in a specialty. I addressed many of their meetings and it was trying to be cooperative, flexible, pleasant whilst having a bottom line and then you would ... reach a crunch point and say you are doing it and a fair few of them came along with me.

Developing good working relationships at all levels and all phases, especially implementation, was explicitly prioritised. Describing one of the joint Chairs, a participant said it was agreed that "we need a really key person who is going to be influential, the status to be able to relate to the sector ... from the point of view of persuasion, influence and mana [or respect from colleagues]." One participant saw this as a consequence of the unique New Zealand approach to primary care: "We don't operate by command and control so ... it is about people and relationships and influence; ... [the NHS] overall system is command and control ... it is a much more strongly medical model than in New Zealand. It is accepted that the doctor will be the leader of the team, whereas, if you said that in New Zealand you would not get out alive."

Design needed to be managed through individuals because "there is not a unified representative structure for general practice ... [and within general practice] you certainly have different groups." One participant, comparing the New Zealand scene with England, found that general practice was "slightly fragmented and doesn't speak with the same political voice that the BMA does." Even the leaders of national organisations agreed that there were major divisions between them as well as between the large organisations and some smaller ones "who weren't part of the national thinking." Another participant says,

> In those days the College was in bed with the government, the NZMA were working as one and the rural general practice network didn't count so much really and then you had [large PHOs] and PHONZ [Primary Health Organisations New Zealand] ... who had a completely different view of the world; ... there was always a tension between Health Care Aotearoa, the Māori-led PHOs and the mainstream white pākehā [New Zealand European] organisations.

Some expressed a view that differences of policy preferences existed between those people considered to be leaders of general practice and the main body of opinion within general practice. It was suggested that leaders were more sensitive to threats to the independence and autonomy of the profession.

The IPAs were a distinct set of interests in the institutional mix. A participant's assessment is that the general practice sector's response to government's introduction of contracting and desire to organise primary health care more systematically, "became dominated by health sector corporates whose membership was private and that were dealing with very large amounts of public money so the dynamic then changed very considerably." As a participant explained, "going from a Union Health Care Clinic to a Procare [a large IPA]—two vastly different structures."

Another participant remembers that:

those big corporates [IPA]—their behaviour was mixed. Quite a lot of it was progressive and pro-system and quite a lot of it was self-interested … basically holding back … [in the face of] government … wanting legitimately to have a say in what goes on in primary care.

One participant characterised the successive attempts by governments over the years to make policy as a "ridiculous dance of 'please do this we are begging you and we will give you a bit of money' and they say 'bugger off'". Another participant noted that the government position on "boundaries between legitimate government control and private sector control" has been confused over the years and subject to debate while the IPAs, for instance, have been much clearer about where those boundaries lay.

## SOLVING THE TECHNICAL CHALLENGES

Technical challenges dominated the design of the PP to a greater extent than the policymaking process in England. Problems relating to choice of indicators and obtaining access to data led to a decision to proceed with implementation on an incremental basis.

### Choice of Indicators

Although a comprehensive set of 29 indicators was proposed by the RSAG in 2002, consultation with the sector failed to achieve agreement on this larger set. A final set of 13 was selected and implemented.

### Obtaining Access to Data

The problems of inadequate centrally accessible data were frequently mentioned by participants as a barrier to the scheme. A Ministry official acknowledged that to move to the stage of more meaningful data would require access to practice management systems which would raise the questions about "ownership of clinical information and its accessibility to people outside practice. That is the next major challenge for the health sector." This was a major issue: it was believed a new database would have taken many years to create (private conversation). A participant saw general practice claiming to "own the data" and although some participants agreed "you needed real time data," another thought this would lead to government seeking to obtain access to practice data using "spyware."

Initial data was in fact drawn from systems designed for payment purposes so presented many quality problems to the implementation team.

This differs from the situation in England where policymakers were able to rapidly design and implement a new computerised database to give real-time feedback to practices on progress towards targets. As in England, the route to data access and increased clinical accountability in New Zealand lay through the profession, which held information critical to a large and adequately monitored set of targets, though it existed in a variety of largely unconnected databases. In the New Zealand case study the profession can be seen to be using patient data-management systems as a source of power, contending that they owned the data and therefore had a key strategic advantage over the operation of the whole system. One participant believed that they would drive a very hard bargain for access to the data. An effect of this strategy was dramatically to limit the PP in scope. Without the engagement of the profession as a whole in the negotiation of an agreement to share detailed information about general practice activities on a national basis, the scheme was bound to be limited, having a reduced potential impact upon health outcomes.

### *Testing the Model*

Scepticism about pay-for-performance, coupled with recognition of the imperfect levers and limited history of effective accountability mechanisms between the state funders and general practice, drove the decision to proceed cautiously with pay-for-performance. A participant says the Ministry believed that "being able to evolve it rather than a revolution was quite important" and officials wished to evolve it as they could see it working. Several participants commented upon the anxiety felt about pay-for-performance schemes having unintended consequences ("the amount of money was small because of nervousness … it could be increased over time if it proved to be effective"; it was a "building towards equity, quality and better outcomes"). Some note that the QOF was being closely watched and "our people were happier with [small incentive money] because they felt that … there is a risk it will take you down too narrow a pathway." Pay-for-performance could be "oversold" according to one participant, seeing it as "one piece of the jig saw but only one piece…. What does it take to influence clinical decision-making—the environment in which you work, your contact with peers, focus groups, measurement, reward for measurement? But it isn't a silver bullet."

## EVALUATIONS AND REVIEWS OF THE PP

In 2008 the organisation responsible for implementing the PP commissioned an evaluation of the PP which was published in December that year (Martin Jenkins & Associates Ltd. 2008). Although most PHOs saw the PP indicators as offering a narrow but reasonable snapshot of best practice, they tended to qualify this with the view that the indicators are partial or less important indicators of quality practice and risked diversion of effort from other more pressing clinical matters. There was dispute about the fairness of the performance framework.

Evaluators found that visibility of the PP was highest among management rather than clinical staff. Correspondingly, many management staff did not know what clinical staff did with the data from the PP when they received it, the processes of clinical leadership and peer support for clinicians being separate from management of the PHO. Various funding allocation practices existed, with two of the six PHOs not distributing performance payments and most sharing these between the PHOs and practices. Data exchange and distribution caused a variety of concerns relating to confidence in its quality, the privacy of the data exchange process and timing of reporting periods (feedback of performance under the scheme was delayed by several months after the end of the reporting period). In this relatively small sample of PHOs, general practitioners received feedback reports mainly from practice managers in a process of administrative feedback rather than peer-led debate and critique of practice.

The evaluators found that the impact of the PP on clinical quality supported this in a low-profile way rather than driving practice improvement itself. It reflected achievements rather than incentivised them, and the primary reward was evidence of improved quality, not payment.

This feedback confirms the significant difference in the mode of operation of incentives in the scheme by contrast to the English scheme, targeted as they are in the PP on the actions of primary care organisations rather than the actions of individual general practitioners. The scheme did not directly incentivise the health actions of individual practitioners in the same way as the QOF did in England. The evaluators concluded that the heterogeneity of the PHO and practice landscape and the separation of management and clinical roles provided considerable challenges to the PP's effectiveness. Future success in achieving clinical behaviour change would be dependent upon PHOs obtaining greater leverage with clinicians, the availability of reliable credible and timely data and the role of champions.

The evaluation indicates some fundamental flaws in the design of the scheme if it is assessed as an incentive scheme to change health actions or the day-to-day decision of general practitioners. Against this criterion it has many shortcomings by comparison with the QOF.

The PP was evaluated further in 2012 (Cranleigh Health 2012), comprehensively reviewing its strategic vision and purpose, its impact on service planning and delivery and its information technology systems and impact on data capture. This evaluation found that the sector saw the PP as a valuable programme, was the only programme that rewards activity on a performance basis and was widely seen as a potential vehicle for future collaborative primary care data development. However, a need for speedier development of indicators and improvements in data integrity and timeliness were expressed. The need for a higher level of incentives to reward efforts to drive results more effectively into high-needs populations (who are harder to reach) was expressed (Cranleigh Health 2012, p. 5).

The evaluation records performance trends for the current set of funded indicators. These had evolved from the initial set to address more pressing population health targets, including ischaemic cardiovascular disease detection and risk assessment, diabetes detection and follow-up, influenza vaccinations of older people and immunisations of children under two (all from 2009) and recording of smoking (from 2010) and advice on smoking cessation (from 2011). Performance against all targets had improved at the PHO level. Performance improvement was more rapid for high-needs populations, and the gap between these and low-needs populations had decreased since 2006. By 2012 the PP had become broadened to include indicators for health actions which had higher potential for a positive impact upon population health outcomes and had results which were reflecting greater levels of quality improvement in services for populations with higher needs. These mirror the results found for the QOF, although in England they were achieved more rapidly.

The evaluation finds there was still mixed support for the PP and rising sector frustration with the low usability and minimal approach to enhancements for data capture and interrogation in practice management systems and the effort required for data collection. Greater transparency and granularity of and access to data was also identified as a major point of dispute, with debates about this causing frustration between stakeholders (such as the Ministry of Health) "seeking greater utilisation, publication and transparency of activity and others, mainly in the primary sector, extremely reluctant to do so" (ibid., p. 24). These problems had been avoided in England with the design and implementation of the QMAS for data capture and reporting.

Opinions differed about whether the PP improved quality of care, with some stakeholders viewing it as setting important clinical governance baselines, others finding it an interference with patient care and others regarding it as "cookbook" medicine.

The governance group for the PP (whose membership gradually expanded) was regarded as reflecting a variety of sectoral interests rather than providing strong leadership, though there was moderate agreement that the advisory committee for the PP had the right clinical experts. At the time 9 of 14 members were from primary care, 3 being practising general practitioners. This had resolved earlier concerns about the "perceived shortage of clinical leadership ... particularly around indicator selection" in the design of the original set of indicators (Martin Jenkins & Associates Ltd. 2008, p. 4).

### Impact on Ambulatory-Sensitive Admissions

It will be seen that in England, evaluators were able to demonstrate a statistically significant association between higher levels of achievement on clinical indicators for coronary heart disease, hypertension, congestive heart failure, diabetes and chronic obstructive pulmonary disease (Dixon 2010, p. 121) and measures of population outcomes such as rates of ambulatory care hospital admissions. Although a reduction in ambulatory-sensitive admissions was not specifically a key measure of success and was used more to motivate reform of existing primary health-care arrangements in presentations about the proposed PHCS, Cranleigh Health utilised this measure in their evaluation and were not able to demonstrate this association in New Zealand for the two of three indicators which might have reasonably been expected to have this outcome (cardiovascular disease [CVD] assessment and detection, influenza vaccinations and immunisations). This is possibly because the indicators were too recently introduced (as is the case with CVD) or the number of hospital admissions for influenza was small. A statistically significant relationship was found between PP achievements for immunisation of children under two and vaccine-preventable hospital admissions (Cranleigh Health 2012, p. 50).

Overall, the ambulatory-sensitive hospital admissions for Māori and Pacific Island peoples had remained the same or increased from 2000/1 to 2005/6 although they declined for non-Māori or non-Pacific Island New Zealanders (Minister of Health 2007, p. 8).

### Review of Performance and Incentive Framework

In 2013 an Expert Advisory Group was convened to recommend a new integrated performance and incentive framework for the health system, which would include primary care. The final report of the Group, published in February 2014, signalled a fundamentally new strategy to address equity, safety, quality, access and cost of services (including unexplained variation of referred services). Comprising nationally set system-level measures and processes for reporting and assessing performance, the framework confers levels of achievement and incentives based on performance on PHOs. However, within national targets, detailed quality improvement measures are developed locally in clinical and consumer-led alliances to reflect local needs. The PP resources are re-directed to provide direct incentive payments to practices which achieve performance targets and to up-front allocations of investment to PHOs to support capability and capacity improvement (Ministry of Health 2014). The framework does not in itself modify other policy settings such as funding, co-payments or service coverage, but substantially re-designs the current PP, incentivising quality improvement at the practice level more directly, with greater potential to influence health actions of practitioners and other practice staff more directly. There is a risk that it will lose the explicit connection between a health action of a general practitioner and the availability of a reward. However the changes may result in greater ability for policymakers to achieve more pronounced associations between general practitioner performance and ambulatory-sensitive hospital admission levels.

### References

Barnett, P., Malcolm, L., Wright, L., & Hendry, C. (2004). Professional Leadership and Organisational Change: Progress Towards Developing a Quality Culture in New Zealand's Health System. *The New Zealand Medical Journal, 117*, 1198.

Barnett, P., Tenbensel, T., Cumming, J., Clayden, C., Ashton, T., Pledger, M., et al. (2009). Implementing New Modes of Governance in the New Zealand Health System: An Empirical Study. *Health Policy, 93*, 118–127.

Crampton, P. (2000). Policies for General Practice. In P. Davis & T. Ashton (Eds.), *Health and Public Policy in New Zealand*. Auckland: Oxford University Press.

Crampton, P., Davis, P., Lay-Yee, R., Raymont, A., Forrest, C., & Starfield, B. (2004). Comparison of Private For-profit with Private Community-Governed Not-for-profit Primary Care Services in New Zealand. *Journal of Health Services Research & Policy, 9*(Suppl 2), 17–22.

Cranleigh Health. (2012). *PHO Performance Programme Evaluation*. Auckland: Cranleigh Health.

Cumming, J., & Mays, N. (2002). Reform and Counter Reform: How Sustainable Is New Zealand's Latest Health System Restructuring? *Journal of Health Services Research & Policy, 7*(Suppl 1), 46–55.

Cumming, J., & Mays, N. (2011). New Zealand's Primary Health Care Strategy: Early Effects of the New Financing and Payment System for General Practice and Future Challenges. *Health Economics, Policy and Law, 6*, 1–21.

Davis, P., Gribben, B., Lay-Yee, R., & Scott, A. (2002). How Much Variation in Clinical Activity Is There Between General Practitioners? A Multi-level Analysis of Decision-Making in Primary Care. *Journal of Health Services Research & Policy, 7*(4), 202–208.

Devlin, N., Maynard, A., & Mays, N. (2001). New Zealand's New Health Sector Reforms: Back to the Future? *BMJ, 322*, 1171–1174.

Dixon, A., Khachatryan, A., Wallace, A., Peckham, S., Boyce, T., & Gillam, S. (2010). *The Quality and Outcomes Framework (QOF): Does It Reduce Health Inequalities?* Final Report. London: National Institute for Health Research.

Finlayson, M. (2000). Policy Implementation and Modification. In P. Davis & T. Ashton (Eds.), *Health and Public Policy in New Zealand*. Auckland: Oxford University Press.

Flood, C. (2001). *Profiles of Six Health Care Systems*. Toronto: University of Toronto.

Gauld, R., & Mays, N. (2006). Are New Zealand's New Primary Health Organsations Fit for Purpose? *BMJ, 333*, 1216–1218.

Gribben, B., Coster, G., Pringle, M., & Simon, J. (2002). Quality of Care Indicators for Population-Based Primary Care in New Zealand. *New Zealand Medical Journal, 115*(1151), 163–166.

Hay, I. (1989). *The Caring Commodity*. Wellington: Oxford University Press.

Hefford, M., Crampton, P., & Foley, J. (2005). Reducing Health Disparities Through Primary Care Reform: The New Zealand Experiment. *Health Policy, 72*, 9–23.

King, A. (2000). *The New Zealand Health Strategy*. Wellington: Ministry of Health.

King, A. (2001). *The Primary Health Care Strategy*. Wellington: Ministry of Health.

Laugesen, M. (2000). The Institutional Context. In P. Davis & T. Ashton (Eds.), *Health and Public Policy in New Zealand*. Auckland: Oxford University Press.

Malcolm, L. (2004). *Peer Review of Referred Services Management Documents*. M. o. Health. Wellington: Aotearoa Health.

Malcolm, L., & Mays, N. (1999a). New Zealand's Independent Practitioner Associations: A Working Model of Clinical Governance in Primary Care? *BMJ*, *319*, 1340–1342.

Malcolm, L., Wright, L., Seers, M., & Guthrie, J. (1999b). An Evaluation of Pharmaceutical Management and Budget Holding in Pegasus Medical Group. *The New Zealand Medical Journal*, *112*, 162–164.

Malcolm, L., Wright, L., & Barnett, P. (2000). Emerging Clinical Governance: Developments in Independent Practitioner Associations in New Zealand. *New Zealand Medical Journal*, *113*, 33–36.

Martin Jenkins & Associates Ltd. (2008). *Evaluation of the PHO Performance Programme*. Wellington.

Mays, N., & Hand, K. (2000). *A Review of Options for Health and Disability Support Purchasing in New Zealand*. Wellington: The Treasury.

Minister of Health. (2007). *The Primary Health Care Strategy—Monitoring Its Achievements 2007: Memo to the Cabinet Social Development Committee*. Wellington: Health.

Ministry of Health. (2005). *PHO Performance Management Programme*. M. o. Health.

Ministry of Health. (2014). *Integrated Performance and Incentive Framework Expert Advisory Group*. Final Report. Health. Wellington: Ministry of Health.

NZLP. (1999). *Labour on Health*. Wellington: New Zealand Labour Party.

O'Malley, C. (2003). *A Reality Check: The Early Sector Response to the Primary Health Care Strategy*. Wellington: Wellington Independent Practitioners Association and Compass Health.

OECD. (2004). *Towards High Performing Health Systems*. Paris: OECD.

Referred Services Advisory Group. (2002). *Referred Services Management: Building Towards Equity, Quality and Better Health Outcomes*. Wellington: Ministry of Health.

Smith, J., & Mays, N. (2007). Primary Care Organisations in New Zealand and England: Tipping the Balance of the Health System in Favour of Primary Care? *International Journal of Health Planning and Management*, *22*, 3–19.

Starke, P. (2010). Why Institutions Are Not the Only Thing That Matters: Twenty-Five Years of Health Care Reform in New Zealand. *Journal of Health Politics, Policy and Law*, *35*(4), 487–516.

Stevens, S. (2004). Reform Strategies for the English NHS. *Health Affairs*, *23*(3), 37–44.

Tuohy, C. H. (1999). *Accidental Logics*. Oxford: Oxford University Press.

# CHAPTER 7

# Utility of Kingdon's Framework: Policymaking in New Zealand

**Abstract** Kingdon's theory that loosely coupled policymaking environments are ripe for exploitation by an exogenous policy entrepreneur is challenged by this New Zealand case study of pay-for-performance policymaking. His hypothesis, that non-incremental change occurs where ambiguity of preferences, fluid participation and unclear technology exist, is partly supported. In a comparative study in which both Kingdon's Multiple Streams Framework and five single-driver theories of policy change are systematically applied to the case study evidence, the Multiple Streams Framework is found to be the most useful. However, it fails to encourage recognition of the powerful institutional and interest group factors or the influence of history at work. Amendments to the Framework reflecting historical antecedents, ownership and governance arrangements, and the role of state-appointed institutional entrepreneurs are recommended.

**Keywords** Multiple Streams Framework • Historical antecedents • Institutionalism • Parliamentary systems • Rational choice drivers

© The Author(s) 2018
V. Smith, *Bargaining Power*,
https://doi.org/10.1007/978-981-10-7602-2_7

## NON INCREMENTAL CHANGE IN CONDITIONS OF AMBIGUITY, FLUID PARTICIPATION AND UNCLEAR TECHNOLOGY?

The introduction of the PP more closely matches Kingdon's definition of non-incremental change than incremental change, although it took longer to implement than the QOF in England. The other conditions which Kingdon suggests will nurture non-incremental change *did* apply in New Zealand. The health sector was an environment of differing, if not exactly ambiguous, policy preferences contending for attention, with considerable fluidity of participation and unclear and inadequate technology for many of the policymaking activities under way at the time. Both committees convened for designing the pay-for-performance programme contained members with a wide variety of views and interests, types of professional expertise and levels of engagement with the policy problem. They were developing policy in an environment of rapidly changing rules and new policy goals. This required much innovation and flexibility in the policymaking process as well as a need to look for existing models which could be quickly adapted for new purposes. Some political uncertainty also existed in 2001 in that the Labour government was halfway through its first term of office and had a history of short periods in office. The situation was, according to Kindgon's model, "loosely coupled" or ripe for political manipulation by a policy entrepreneur (Tuohy 2012, p. 4).

It is important to note that the pay-for-performance policymaking process was operational policymaking nested within a larger strategic policymaking process, the design and implementation of the PHCS, which was also planned, top-down, non-incremental, boldly designed and rapidly enacted and implemented by politicians within the Politics Stream. This overarching reform was intended to achieve a sea change or "counterrevolution" (Gauld 2003; Starke 2010) in the way governance and structural arrangements in the health system, including payment systems for Vote Health funding, worked. Within it, the implementation of the PP followed a different pattern, being subject to extensive consultation and a phased and voluntary process in which many decisions could be taken at the regional level.

In this case study, agenda-setting occurred in a civil servant–led committee. Alternative selection occurred in a new phase of work accomplished through a large committee led by jointly appointed Chairs with a mix of general practice service delivery management and health services funding and development experience.

Although no "classic Kingdon" policy entrepreneur is found in the study (neither is one readily identifiable in the development of the PHCS overarching policymaking process), it can be argued that actors resembling *institutional* entrepreneurs were recruited and made a key contribution during the alternative selection stage of policymaking. These have been described as "exploring the transferable, concealed and dormant institutional resources of their societies" (Crouch 2005, p. 157) and being effective in environments in which uncertainty exists as well as heterogeneity. This is more so when political uncertainty or the inability to predict political shifts could change the landscape for new institutional arrangements (Tuohy 2012, p. 4). This is a particular characteristic of the New Zealand health policymaking environment in which fierce partisan positions, short terms of office and relatively frequent changes of administrations differ somewhat from the English health policymaking environment. This is explored below in the section "Policy Entrepreneurs".

## Problems Stream

This policymaking episode arises in the Problems Stream which, according to Zahariadis, will be more likely to lead to a rational approach to policymaking, as borne out by the evidence. During the implementation phase of the larger PHCS (which created its "policy window"), the problem arose of how to maintain a quality-oriented approach to pharmaceutical and laboratory services use under the new PHCS structures, capitated funding and principles for equity of access and outcomes. An additional policymaking challenge was how to change inequities in prescribing and funding of the services for poorer communities. A mechanism was needed to redistribute resources and rectify variances in prescribing patterns.

Indicators of the need for a new policy included analysis of prescribing patterns showing unexplained variances and lower levels of resource in poorer communities and data which showed significant variance in life expectancy for some citizens, particularly Māori. Focusing events included an identified need for new policy to manage allocation of pharmaceutical and laboratory-testing resources identified in the implementation of the PHCS. Feedback to policymakers showed positive results in changing prescribing patterns through budget management contracts, as did reports that significant public funds had been obtained by IPA through savings achieved in these contracts. This work received a lower priority during this primary health-care policy period due to the major workload of policy issues relating to implementation of the PHCS.

## POLITICS STREAM

Kingdon suggests party ideology, administrative turnover and national mood (the latter including balance of interest group attitudes) are relevant, and the first two factors strongly feature in the evidence. Party ideology that influenced the design included a strong commitment to an accessible, equitable health service, concern over privatisation and profit-making from health care, deep concern over inappropriate and inequitable capture of public funds by IPAs, grievances about the history of relationships with general practitioner representatives and concern over disparity of health outcomes. Services appropriate for Māori and Pacific peoples were a strong commitment. There was also a preference for a strong patient and community voice in health service design and concern about medical dominance of health policy. Administrative or legislative turnover was a key driver incentivising rapid policymaking for Labour, recently elected to a three-year term after nine years out of office and now governing in a strong coalition. Labour politicians were determined to restore the integrity of a national health service. But this also acts as a factor incentivising opposition to the policymaking by other interests. The evidence shows that a major feature in this stream was the strong allegiances between particular political parties, their academic advisors and types of general practice organisations. Kingdon suggests that when there is conflict rather than consensus between interest groups, politicians must determine the balance of support and opposition, indicating the price that will be paid for pushing the idea forward (Kingdon 2010, p. 150). This important calculation is reflected in the inclusion of "balance of interests" in the sub-elements of the Zahariadis model of the Politics Stream.

## POLICY STREAM

The value acceptability, technical feasibility and resource adequacy of the policy idea and these features, as well as the integration of the policy community, are all considered by Zahariadis as important sub-elements in the Policy Stream.

**Policy idea:** Pay-for-performance was a controversial idea, attracting some strong negative opinion and academic analysis from some quarters. Improving the quality of general practice was, however, readily accepted as a policy idea. As in England, there were existing budget management and clinical governance initiatives which could be used as templates to develop a national programme for incentivising quality improvement and clinical governance in general practice. But unlike in England these were not nationally consistent, centrally driven or underpinned by the new values of equitable redistribution of resources. The existing initiatives formed a heterogeneous collection of regional initiatives and many distributed their savings to privately owned companies. The policymaking process needed to deliver a nationally consistent framework oriented to equity and population health goals from this heterogenous mix. There was strong academic interest and support from general practice consortia, including the IPAs, for continuation of existing approaches (who depended upon these for an income stream). Many participants in the design process had direct experience of such programmes.

Value acceptability included strong state support for population-based and preventive health practices. Officials were open to new contractual approaches, payment methods and other technical approaches to public sector performance management in order to achieve equity goals. But the scepticism about the merits of pay-for-performance within the bureaucracy, academia and the medical profession was enhanced by the fact that its technical feasibility was a major problem. The state had a new mechanism for enrolling patients with a PHO and these organisations were newly established, with differing capacity and capability to develop or influence existing clinical governance systems, few existing national practice or quality frameworks, minimal availability of national databases suitable for a performance programme and a regionalised structure for implementing the policy.

**Policy community:** The evidence reveals that there were low levels of integration of the general practice policy community, especially on the subject of quality systems and governance arrangements. There were differing levels of access to politicians and civil service decision-makers held by different types of organisations. Access often depended on political allegiances of the organisations. Competitive modes of discourse and adversarial decision-making processes were often used between stakeholders in the policy community and there were variable levels of organisational and administrative capacity among organisations. There was a limited history or track record of policymaking partnerships between the general practice profession and state actors. To reiterate, a partisan pattern existed, which broadly saw community-based groups working with Labour and private general practice interests working with the National Party.

## POLICY WINDOW

The policy window included a coupling logic which was consequential on a need arising as part of implementation of the PHCS as well as doctrinal. DHBs urgently required a process to assist them to redistribute prescribing and laboratory referral funding more equitably and achieve more equitable use of the funds—and the Labour Party had a doctrinal commitment to equitable distribution of resources and services. The decision style was bold for the larger overarching policymaking but very cautious for its implementation and for the policymaking which arose from its implementation.

## POLICY ENTREPRENEURS

According to Kingdon's MS Framework, conditions were optimal for a policy entrepreneur to emerge and manipulate this policymaking situation. No visible policy entrepreneur was identified as Kingdon's classic "power brokers who manipulate problematic preferences and unclear technology and exploit the system's fluid participation rates to push forth their pet solutions" (Zahariadis 2003, p. 520). Civil servants set the agenda for the policy, with advice from academics, as they implemented the manifesto commitments of the Labour government. This process was overseen by traditional Cabinet government processes more clearly than was the policymaking process in England, where the "sofa cabinet" style of policymaking was practised.

As in England, the issues of access, resources and strategies are not relevant to this case study because the policymaking was officially mandated. This case study is an example of strong civil service leadership and management of the policymaking process. Few strategies such as framing, affect priming or symbols were used, but salami tactics or piece-by-piece tactics were deliberately employed during the implementation phase to minimise disruption, test the model and build support.

However in the alternative selection phase, entrepreneurial actors were deliberately recruited, fitting the description of institutional entrepreneurs as developed by Crouch (2005), and these actors helped develop new forms of governance, including clinical governance, for the new PHOs. One of the major policy challenges from these health reforms was to build capacity within primary health-care organisations to understand and work within a capitated funding allocation and deliver population-based preventive health-care services. Actors who had been involved in their own regional initiatives to introduce capitation funding and quality improvement systems in the 1990s were institutional entrepreneurs, able to draw on their own experiences of innovations in such approaches. General practitioners who had experiences of working in capitated funding environments or in Māori and Pacific communities were particularly important in the debate over the design of the scheme, effectively placing their professional expertise and credibility as clinicians at the service of both funders and their profession. They exhibited attributes of social acuity, team-building and leadership by example. Because of the small, incremental, regionalised, low-profile and voluntary nature of the scheme they consequently faced fewer reputational or public support risks than the English policymakers, and the policy design process generally held few political risks. However, leaders of the policymaking process recruited from general practice faced reputational risks such as loss of professional standing and influence within those parts of the professional community which opposed the pay-for-performance policy and its policymaking process and with politicians from opposing parties who did not support a community-led approach to governance of primary health-care services. As in England, therefore, the greatest risks faced by the institutional entrepreneurs arose from those that might arise in the event of a change in government and the conditions upon which they had based their strategy.

## MOTIVATION OF ENTREPRENEURS

The evidence provides some insight into the motivations and strategies of the institutional entrepreneurs who led the design of the PP in its alternative selection stage. They wished to balance strong personal commitments to reduce inequalities with the desire to reward quality and support clinical governance (having a track record of championing a capitation-based approach to primary health-care funding as the most appropriate vehicle to do this). They were very committed to achieving a balanced consultative forum, to build consensus for the features of the PP and to get ownership for the new pay-for-performance policy. They wished to manage or reduce the divisions within the general practice community and reduce the tensions between Labour politicians and some sections of that community. They were strongly committed to broadening the multi-disciplinary approaches to primary care service delivery through team-based, not doctor-dominated, practices.

The evidence suggests they were willing to risk professional standing and influence due to their policymaking activities for the social purpose which animated them, in particular taking forward the inequalities agenda to ensure that Māori and poorer communities had improved access to higher quality primary health care. The same motivation, though not the same risk, was observed among the civil servants charged with the initial design, who made comments that disadvantaged populations were "missing out" as a rationale for putting "much more focus on equity."

### Explanatory Comprehensiveness of Kingdon's MS Framework

To recap, non-incremental change, in Kingdon's definition, was achieved in the New Zealand health reforms. The scale and pace of change was determined by the Executive. The case study displays the differences between the two policymaking activities during this period: the overarching health system policymaking, a significant non-incremental change, was rapidly implemented and had closely managed participation and clear technology for implementation (it was straightforward to introduce governance changes such as restoring the District Health Boards for instance); and the pay-for-performance policymaking episode which was also non-incremental but had more signs of ambiguity, fluid participation and unclear technology, and a phased, more consultative, regionalised and slower implementation process. This reflected pragmatic realities of policymaking in the general practice sub-system with its multiple forms of governance and ownership of primary care services, many contending interests and few integrating information systems or antecedent national quality improvement policies, such as existed in England, which could be built upon. Although conditions were suitable for a classic Kingdon exogenous policy entrepreneur to operate as part of the pay-for-performance policymaking episode (given the ambiguity of preferences and the clear policy window), this did not happen. Endogenous actors with entrepreneurial skills, as in England, were recruited to help develop new decision-making and governance systems to support the new policies designed by civil servants and politicians, assist in changes of institutions, as well as with policies to support greater public accountability in general practices.

## OTHER DRIVERS OF POLICYMAKING PROCESSES

Based on the analysis above, there are some major gaps in the way the model captures and encourages us to look for key drivers and features of the policymaking process which were, in the empirical research undertaken for this study, shown to be critical to the policymaking episode. These are now set out below.

### *Institutional Features*

The institutional sub-system for general practice in New Zealand which structured the relationship between the state and interest group actors, as in England, is a critical variable in this episode. The history of health policymaking in New Zealand had led to the following features:

- a heterogeneous set of ownership and governance arrangements for general practice service delivery;
- disengagement between Labour politicians and the largest organisations representing general practitioners;
- multiple payer financing arrangements for general practice;
- new arm's-length contractual arrangements for primary care funding which needed to be developed by a large number of newly formed primary care organisations;
- a re-centralised structure for health policymaking, with preferences for regional implementation;
- no representative body for general practice.

Politicians preferred top-down, rationalist and technically driven approaches for initial policy design and delivered the initial civil-service-designed, rapidly developed and comprehensive pay-for-performance proposal. Then a cautious, consultative and stakeholder-oriented approach to alternative selection and policy implementation of the pay-for-performance framework followed.

This pattern, described by Tuohy as "big bang" change characteristic of Westminster adversarial systems reflects the different facilitators, barriers and trajectories for policymaking from those seen in governing systems with federal structures or a separation of powers (Tuohy 2012, p. 12).

Finlayson's characterisation of the implementation phase in New Zealand as not a "neutral non-political stage of the policymaking process … especially where key groups have not been involved in the formulation of policy" (Finlayson 2000), describes the risks of these dynamics in this country. The evidence shows that the new Labour government had learned from the troubles of the previous administration in the implementation phase for its primary health-care policies and sought to minimise these by some more-extended use of strategic alliances and stakeholder management strategies, albeit within the terms of an uncompromising policy stance on a community-led governance model.

The institutional features of the general practice sub-system and the recent history of failed attempts to implement major health policy change vindicated this cautious approach to implementation of the pay-for-performance policy developed by the RSAG, which slowed and regionalised implementation so that it extended over four more years. Even so the process of alternative selection and implementation was unable to solve key design challenges such as general practitioners' buy-in to a broader and more relevant set of population health targets for the scheme or to develop solutions to the information management deficits which limited the scheme to a small set of targets.

Although the intention of the PP was to establish leverage for the new PHOs to influence and support clinical governance frameworks among their general practices, evaluations show that the performance incentives did not always act as drivers of practice change but, as in England, often reflected existing behaviours. Implementation patterns were as heterogenous as the environment into which they were introduced. Clinical governance activities in some primary health organisations remained sequestered within the existing peer-led and collegial systems which New Zealand general practitioners had developed over the years. Some PHO management staff had limited knowledge of or involvement in these processes, at least initially. These institutional features, and the barriers which they placed in the way of the design and implementation of a single large national scheme, delayed and limited the achievement of a new focus on population health and preventive practices and any potential for improvements in health outcomes.

## Heterogeneity of the Institutional Landscape

Considering the two case study analyses together, the differences between the impact of a heterogenous institutional landscape in the general practice sub-system in New Zealand and the more homogenous, centrally coordinated landscape in England become clearer. This makes the nature of the institutional landscape a strong candidate as a driver of difference in the size, scope and speed of policy design.

New Zealand's heterogeneous environment, with large elements disaffected in some ways from the government's policies for primary health care, meant that the process of alternative selection and implementation of the new policy had to be carefully planned if it was not to falter, as had been the case with earlier health policy implementation attempts in the 1990s. It also affected technical feasibility of implementation. A practical consequence of the widespread lack of collaboration or engagement with the new policy was the problem of data adequacy. Existing national databases held information on only a small number of activities which could be suitable for development as pay-for-performance targets. Processes designed for the selection of new indicators were unwieldy and time-consuming and participants withdrew from these. It was not considered feasible to implement an information management system to support a real-time feedback mechanism on practice activity and performance such as the QMAS. A feature of the New Zealand scheme was that the calculation of results and payment of incentives was delayed by 6–12 months after each achievement period. This further deterred general practitioner engagement.

Devolved implementation also slowed progress. PHOs varied in their capacity and capability to implement the PP. Whereas in England implementation occurred at the practice level by practices eager to demonstrate performance and release new income, in New Zealand implementation depended upon the readiness of both District Health Boards and PHOs and the central PP team. These organisations had many other pressing priorities for their resources and attention from 2006 to 2008 (including implementation of major immunisation and other population health-related campaigns). Some features such as the variation in amounts of payments for performance and the ease and speed with which practices obtained feedback about their performance under the scheme differed widely. Where these were perceived as unfair or inadequate, practices were less interested in participating in the PP (Martin Jenkins & Associates Ltd.

2008). However, devolved implementation permitted the building of local or regional coalitions around the new policy to reflect local conditions, needs and preferences and contributed to its longevity through successive administrations.

### *Historical Antecedents*

The evidence shows that historical events, relationships and policies influenced policymaking processes. The genesis of the national health system and the relationship between the Labour Party, in and out of office, and parts of the medical profession in New Zealand is an ever-present theme in the minds of most participants interviewed about the process of policy design. Because of this history, feelings ran high among some participants. Opposition politicians were subsequently cultivated by the Independent Practitioners' Association Council to champion different approaches to clinical leadership. The evidence points to some participants deciding to bide their time until a change of government would enable them to exercise greater influence and redress the policy design in their favour.

The existence of antecedents of the quality improvement and budget management schemes developed by general practice consortia, including IPAs, a decade earlier were critical to facilitating the design of this scheme. Personnel involved in these earlier schemes were heavily involved in designing the new one and used their experience from these schemes in their work. Evidence about the need for and effectiveness of such policies in academic studies of the impacts of the early budget management schemes was used in making the case for and designing the scheme.

## DOES THE ZAHARIADIS MODEL ENCOURAGE CONSIDERATION OF THESE FACTORS?

While the model is very helpful in providing five structural elements which display key features of the policymaking process in New Zealand it does not go far enough to highlight certain elements which have been found to be important influencers of the process. The set of sub-elements in the Zahariadis model does not invite specific consideration of interest group institutional structure or underpinning ownership and governance features which may influence or explain these interest group attributes. It does not invite consideration of the type of policymaking which is incentivised by different electoral and governing systems. It does not consider forms of institutional entrepreneurial behaviour which are focused upon the building of new governance or decision-making systems rather than on new policies.

## REFERENCES

Crouch, C. (2005). *Capitalist Diversity and Change*. Oxford: Oxford University Press.

Finlayson, M. (2000). Policy Implementation and Modification. In P. Davis & T. Ashton (Eds.), *Health and Public Policy in New Zealand*. Auckland: Oxford University Press.

Gauld, R. (2003). One Country, Four Systems: Comparing Changing Helath Policies in New Zealand. *International Political Science Review, 24*(2), 199–218.

Kingdon, J. W. (2010). *Agendas, Alternatives, and Public Policies, Update Edition, with an Epilogue on Health Care*. London: Longmans.

Martin Jenkins & Associates Ltd. (2008). *Evaluation of the PHO Performance Programme*. Wellington.

Starke, P. (2010). Why Institutions Are Not the Only Thing That Matters: Twenty-Five Years of Health Care Reform in New Zealand. *Journal of Health Politics, Policy and Law, 35*(4), 487–516.

Tuohy, C. H. (2012). *Institutional Entrepreneurs and the Politics of Redesigning the Welfare State: The Case of Health Care*. New Orleans, a paper to be presented at the annual meeting of the American Political Science Association, New Orleans, Louisiana.

Zahariadis, N. (2003). Ambiguity and Choice in European Public Policy. *Journal of European Public Policy, 15*(4), 514–530.

# CHAPTER 8

# The Two Case Studies Compared

**Abstract** Bargaining power is shown to be the driver of non-incremental policy change and variation in a thought-provoking comparative analysis of two health policymaking case studies. England's policymakers were able to integrate a pay-for-performance scheme design into contractual negotiations with the British Medical Association, leading to increased funder influence over general practitioners and opportunities to improve population health outcomes. Contemporaneously, New Zealand's policymakers lacked these powers, delivering a much smaller scheme. Kingdon's Multiple Streams Framework fails to offer adequate explanations for the policymaking in these two majoritarian, parliamentary political systems. Recommendations are made for modifications to the Framework to recognise the importance of institutional context in the Politics Stream, variation in entrepreneurial activity and policy outcomes (not just outputs).

**Keywords** Pay-for-performance • Multiple Streams Framework • Bargaining • Majoritarian parliamentary systems • Policy outcomes

Table 8.1 compares the two policymaking processes according to the five main drivers of policy change and their policy outputs and outcomes.

© The Author(s) 2018
V. Smith, *Bargaining Power*,
https://doi.org/10.1007/978-981-10-7602-2_8

**Table 8.1**   The two case studies compared: drivers analysis for pay-for-performance policymaking

| Driver | England | New Zealand |
|---|---|---|
| Institutional | Majoritarian, unitary political system<br>National health system<br>Single-payer GP financing (primarily capitation)<br>Single NHS/GP ownership/ governance model<br>Strong hierarchical corporatist features of decision-making in GP sub-system | Majoritarian, unitary political system<br>National health system<br>Multiple-payer GP financing (primarily fee for service)<br>Multiple GP ownership/governance models<br>Collegial/market features of decision-making in GP sub-system |
| Networks | Integrated GP policy community<br>Single representative GP body<br>BMA holds mandated bargaining rights<br>BMA has high level of access to state actors<br>"Politics of the double bed" history<br>Active well-established medico-academic research community | Heterogeneous GP policy community<br>Multiple representative GP bodies<br>No mandated bargaining rights for GPs<br>Partisan patterns of access to state actors<br>Adversarial history between some GPs and the Labour Party<br>Smaller medico-academic research community |
| Actors | Prime Minister involved in health policy<br>Reforming Secretary of State for Health<br>Executive led policy agenda-setting<br>Civil servants side-lined in policy development<br>Policy design dominated by GPs<br>GP negotiators accountable to GPC/BMA<br>All GPs held vote on final scheme/ contract<br>Policy design led by appointed negotiators. Academics mediated policy design process<br>Insider knowledge/relationship management skills, "policy entrepreneur" experience of practice-based pay-for-performance (p-for-p) scheme used | Prime Minister involved in health policy<br>Reforming Minister of Health<br>Executive endorsed pay-for-performance policy<br>Civil servants led policy agenda-setting<br>GPs minority in policy design teams<br>No GP accountability framework for policy<br>Community-based and other primary care professionals involved in design<br>Policy design led by appointed leaders to develop new governance mechanisms.<br>Insider knowledge/relationship management skills and "institutional entrepreneur" experience of quality improvement in capitated funding environments used |

(*continued*)

**Table 8.1**   (continued)

| Driver | England | New Zealand |
|---|---|---|
| Ideas | NPM-intensive history of public policy | NPM-intensive history of public policy |
| | Government keen to empower primary care | Government keen to empower primary care, community voices and Māori and Pacific communities |
| | Concerned about health inequalities | Concerned about health inequalities |
| | p-for-p trialled in several precursor schemes | P-for-P trialled in several precursor schemes |
| | Strong GP support for fund-holding for hospital services | Strong GP support for budget-holding for referred services |
| | GP scepticism about population-based health | GP scepticism about population-based health |
| | GP scepticism about customer service | Strong GP focus on customer service |
| | Strong commitment to free primary care | Strong commitment to patient co-payment among most GPs |
| | Supportive of centralised quality standards | Limited exposure to central standards |
| | Majority GP support p-for-p and monitoring of practice data in exchange for more income | Support for peer-led utilisation review but many GPs opposed to funder access to data |
| Socio-economic | High predicted burden of chronic conditions | High predicted burden of chronic conditions |
| | Willing to invest more money in primary care | Willing to invest more money in primary care |
| Policy output | Voluntary national pay-for-performance scheme | Voluntary national pay-for-performance scheme |
| | 146 indicators | 13 indicators |
| | Clinical/service domains incentivised | Clinical domains incentivised |
| | 25–30 per cent of income conditional | 2 per cent of income conditional |
| | 1-yr implementation period | 3-yr implementation period |
| | Provision for review of indicators | Provision for review of indicators |

(*continued*)

**Table 8.1**    (continued)

| Driver | England | New Zealand |
|---|---|---|
| Policy outcome | 95 per cent compliance with targets in first year<br>Ambulatory-sensitive admissions impact on:<br>• Coronary heart disease<br>• Hypertension<br>• Congestive heart failure<br>• Diabetes<br>• COPD<br>Choice of indicators in subsequent years undertaken by National Institute of Clinical Excellence<br>By 2014, reduction to 10 per cent of pay conditional on achievement of targets | 81 per cent compliance with targets in first year<br>Ambulatory-sensitive admissions impact on:<br>• Vaccination-related admissions<br>Choice of indicators in subsequent years undertaken by governance group with larger number of GPs<br>By 2014, proposal to review scheme, providing quality-building grants to PHOs and direct incentives to practices for achievement of targets |

## WHAT OUTCOMES WERE ACHIEVED BY THESE POLICYMAKING PROCESSES?

The policy outcomes can be viewed as administrative or health outcomes. Administrative (or stewardship) outcomes describe the ability of the state to better hold general practice to account for its health actions. Health outcomes describe improved health status derived from incentivised changes in practice-based activities. Both types of outcomes differed in each jurisdiction.

### Administrative Outcomes

With respect to administrative outcomes, both policymaking episodes delivered enhancements to each government's ability to set priorities, monitor performance and hold to account providers in the general practice sector. Though more rapid progress towards improved health outcomes was made through England's QOF than through New Zealand's PP, arguably the greater shift in stewardship capability occurred in the New Zealand policymaking episode, given the very low base from which the state needed to develop improved accountability frameworks for general practice. This broader programme included introduction of contracts for primary health-care services, capitated funding allocations, enrolment of patients with PHOs, restoration of universal subsidies and initiatives to redistribute levels of primary care resources according to health need.

**English achievements:** The introduction of the QOF contributed major enhancements to the state's ability to exercise its purchasing functions by incentivising 146 targets for general practitioners to improve population health. Through the policymaking episode, the commissioning function of the state was enhanced to deliver better information systems to record patient health status (through the QMAS) and to monitor what activities were directed, within general practices, to addressing these health needs. The contract was redesigned to place over 25 per cent of general practice income at risk if the required activities were not performed, while preserving the core viability of practice income. These were strong new levers to influence health actions of general practitioners.

Many features of these commissioning, purchasing and contracting arrangements could be improved (Comptroller and Auditor General 2010). There were clear benefits for primary care in England from the introduction of the QOF and other features of the new General Medical Services contract, which improved the retention of general practitioners and increased its attractiveness as a choice of practice within medicine, at least in the years immediately following implementation of the new contract. However, this was at the expense of resources in fiscal and human health services generally, as the contract caused over-spending and excessive recruitment to the general practice sector for some years. Productivity did not increase as a result of the contract, given the higher-than-expected earnings and reduced working hours for general practitioners (Comptroller and Auditor General 2008).

Evaluations of the overall effect of the English contract show mixed results, with general practices in poorer areas lifting their performance more rapidly than in better-off areas in the first years after implementation of the contract (McDonald 2010). More practitioners were attracted to work in all areas, increasing service capacity. But needs-adjusted redistribution of funding generally moved at a slower pace than intended and there were many criticisms of the widespread withdrawal of general practices from after-hours services, with those services replaced by contracted general practice clinics. Some of these issues have been addressed in subsequent negotiations between the government and the profession. Equity risks relating to access barriers (geographic or service-related such as cultural appropriateness) and differential health outcomes remain but evaluators consider that these have been reduced by the QOF.

**New Zealand achievements:** The small number of targets and the low level of engagement of key general practice leaders in the design process initially delivered a smaller enhancement to administrative ability to monitor and influence general practice in New Zealand. While implementation was well managed in the network of PHOs and especially by the central team managing the Performance Plan itself, an "implementation gap" occurred, with many general practitioners not engaging with the PP initially. However, new national information management systems have developed around the PP, showing the relative performance of regions in reaching the PP targets. There is no shared national database of practice activity on the QMAS model though there are services which offer sampling of a representative national practice information dataset for research purposes. After some years the governance of the PP was restructured to incorporate more representatives from general practice, though this slowed the development of targets and indicators for a time. The number of indicators has remained relatively static though the types of indicators have moved towards those more obviously associated with health status such as cardiovascular disease risk assessment, diabetes detection and follow-up, and smoking cessation advice. The policy emphasis on population health and inequalities is seen to have receded with the election of a new government in 2008 (Tenbensel 2011, p. 252). Subsequently, fund reductions were made for the PP; total funding fell from $33 million in 2010 to $21 million in 2011 (PHO Performance Programme 2010, 2011), and there is currently a plan to dismantle the PP in its current form and disperse some of its resources to PHOs for capacity-building initiatives relating to quality and a new Integrated Performance and Incentive Framework (Ministry of Health 2014). The funding position of the state in general practice has also declined as levels of co-payments have gradually increased again. In February 2014 the average fee for an adult to attend a general practice was $31.93 and for a child over six was $22.70.[1]

Some shifts in the nature of governance and accountability dynamics between state actors and the profession were detected by commentators in the years following the election of a National government in 2008. Greater clinician involvement, or "sideways" accountability, particularly in the running of hospitals, was advocated by the new Minister of Health in preference to "downwards" accountability to the community

(Tenbensel 2011). New "Alliance Agreements" have been put into place between funders and providers which aim to reflect a high trust, low bureaucracy environment with high quality and accountability and which are designed to provide a mechanism for clinical leadership in the development of health services.

## Health Outcomes

Potential for health system impact in incentivising more preventive, population-based activities in primary care in each country was high. Recent evaluations of each scheme report levels of statistically significant associations between the pay-for-performance scheme and measures of health outcomes, such as rates of ambulatory care admissions. Although the results are somewhat equivocal (and it should be noted that the reduction of ambulatory-sensitive admissions was not an agreed measure of success of these schemes) these show that England achieved gains in five of the key chronic illnesses (coronary heart disease, hypertension, congestive heart failure, diabetes and chronic obstructive pulmonary disease) while New Zealand achieved this solely for vaccination-related admissions (Dixon 2010; Cranleigh Health 2012).

Studies of the impact of financial incentives on health care rarely report the outcomes of incentive schemes (Saltman 2005). The evaluations of the outcomes of these two schemes provide important feedback for policymakers about their effectiveness and have enabled this comparative research to include an assessment of not only the process and outputs but also the outcomes of both schemes.

## THE STRENGTH OF THE COMPARATIVE CASE

The comparative approach can give greater methodological assurance that the differences between the two case studies did not occur by chance if it can be shown that the two countries are alike in all respects but one or two variables in a "most similar" or "concomitant variation" strategy case study design (Przeworski 1970, pp. 32–33). This most-similar systems case study design, studying matched policymaking processes, has allowed many features to be controlled for, which could be expected to be drivers of policy variation.

According to the logic of the "most similar" strategies, if some important differences are found among these countries then "the number of factors attributed to these differences will be sufficiently small to warrant explanation in terms of those differences alone ... Common systemic characteristics are conceived as controlled for and inter-systemic differences are viewed as explanatory variables." Statements of explanatory variables can be formulated at the sub-systemic level such as each country's general practice sector. Deductive logic is then applied to make the case for these explanatory variables.

In a framework suggested by John (1998, p. 89) the policy outcome is the dependent variable and all other variables are included in the analysis, including those relating to institutions, rational choice explanations, group structure and resources, socio-economic drivers and ideas. The comparative analysis of the New Zealand and English governing systems and their overarching national health systems demonstrates extensive common systemic characteristics. These are therefore controlled for and the inter-systemic differences—namely the general practice institutional features (financing arrangements and ownership and governance structures as well as the relative strength of general practitioner representative associations) which permitted bargaining in one case study—are the explanatory variables.

### Similarities Which Are Relevant to the Case Studies

The case for the common systemic characteristics includes remarkable similarities between the two countries in many respects:

- timing—occurring contemporaneously at the end of a period of neo-liberal government;
- ideology—initiated by social democratic governments with a strong public mandate for investment in health services;
- setting—in similar Westminster model parliamentary systems (though New Zealand had introduced proportional representation, the Labour/Alliance government of 1999 had a large majority);
- similar health reform history—both governments faced a change-weary community of health stakeholders who had previously succeeded in opposing the implementation of legislation, so were equally cautious about the proposed nature and extent of health policy change;
- a broad current of public opinion–supported improvements in health service delivery;

- both pay-for-performance policies had strong continuity with policies from the previous era, especially general practice fund-holding and budget management;
- both are nested within larger health policy reform efforts;
- the medical profession was highly influential in each country;
- good reasons (relating to efficiency, equity and cost-containment) to justify implementing greater accountability within general practice for the delivery of medical services;
- new money was available.

The same goals for primary health care underpinned the purpose of the two policy pay-for-performance initiatives. These include intentions to:

- incentivise general practice-based health actions which prevent or improve the management of chronic health conditions;
- shift resources to under-doctored or under-serviced areas;
- encourage new approaches to workforce utilisation;
- maintain the momentum for greater accountability of health providers to funders created by the health reforms of the 1990s;
- avoid open conflict or imposition of settlements on unwilling parties;
- avoid the risks of pay-for-performance policies by building-in of provisions for review and refinement of targets, mechanisms and funding levels over time.

Both countries built on existing New Public Management-generated policies post 2000 in a way described as a "logic of escalation" (Pollitt 2008) or a dynamic in which an initial tendency for "a few simple measures to become a more comprehensive package" exists. Career civil servants in both countries carried these approaches from one administration to the next and in New Zealand were the primary agenda-setters of the pay-for-performance policy.

### *Differences Relevant to the Case Studies*

These are:

- use of bargaining and negotiation mechanism for developing the pay-for-performance policy;

- institutional/structural framework for general practice sub-system;
- history of relationships between the state and general practice interest group.

The framework for sole bargaining rights in England is a product of history and of the singular ownership and governance structures in the general practice sub-system in that country. It has given rise to a more integrated general practice interest group in England and creates the opportunity and incentive for general practitioners to exercise their bargaining power collectively, through a single democratic representative channel. It is reasonable to conclude that the bargaining framework is an artefact of the institutional arrangements for general practice services, particularly the financing arrangements. Similar institutional and financing arrangements were originally legislated for in New Zealand at the time of health system establishment but diverged markedly over time to produce a multi-payer and heterogeneous context for policymaking without a legitimated bargaining agent. In England the single-payer/single-contract arrangement has been uninterrupted since 1948 and has encouraged the development of a single point of interface for the general practice profession with the state, the BMA.

This leads to the conclusion that the response of each government to the conditions in its general practice sub-system was in fact a rational approach which accorded with the instruments of governance and influence available to them. Whereas in England more direct forms of incentives, focused on the unit of the general practice itself, could be bargained for nationally and achieved more rapidly, in New Zealand a population-based approach to improving primary health care needed to be developed first within its new community-governed PHOs.

## UTILITY OF MS FRAMEWORK

### *Incremental or Non-incremental Change?*

The analysis shows that the English case study exhibits non-incremental change *without* the expected features of ambiguity, fluidity of participation and unclear technology. By contrast the New Zealand case study exhibits much of this ambiguity, fluidity of participation and unclear technology. It delivers change which meets Kingdon's definition of non-incremental change but is smaller in size, scope and speed of implementation.

## Ambiguity, Fluidity and Unclear Technology?

Against the criteria of ambiguity, fluidity and unclear technology, the English and New Zealand case studies deliver contradictory findings. In England where non-incremental change occurred there is planned, top-down policymaking featuring clarity of preferences, closed participation and clear technology for implementation. The evidence shows that ambiguity, fluidity and unclear technology do apply to the New Zealand case study, which also delivers non-incremental change, but with a step-by-step process of implementation.

The two case studies reinforce the conclusion that policymaking in Westminster systems can be planned, top-down and non-incremental in purposeful and orderly circumstances, that political leaders do indeed make decisions about the scale and pace of change and these strategies reflect the political and institutional settings in which they operate. This leads to a question about the importance of the entrepreneurial role itself and Kingdon's theory of political manipulation. The case studies show that it was not at the agenda-setting phase that these actors were important. During this phase in Westminster systems, political parties and ministers dominate. At the subsequent stages of alternative selection and implementation, however, other actors including civil servants and entrepreneurial actors play a much more significant role.

## Importance of Policy Entrepreneurs

In both case studies, the exogenous manipulative policy entrepreneur is not found but actors with a variety of entrepreneurial skills are seen to be enlisted by governments to bring disparate ideas together to explore common ground and to conciliate different interests. Policy change in each case study was facilitated by individual actors exhibiting entrepreneurial skills as described in the MS Framework literature. However, this evidence does not add up to a theory of political manipulation at the agenda-setting phase. These actors are most relevant in the alternative selection phase though were acting according to the directions of ministers.

These actors can be seen as entrepreneurial because they "gamble that certain resources can be combined now to yield greater value at some uncertain future state than they do in their current use" (Tuohy 2012, p. 1). They assisted state funders to enter into clinical debates with general practitioners, without directly challenging the professional autonomy of general practitioners, enabling the state to influence the use of health resources by medical professionals. They carried out this public mandate by combining the authority of the state with their specialised knowledge (Tuohy 2012, p. 3) and their previous experience of such innovations at the regional level.

So in summary, actors utilising entrepreneurial skills were important to the successful conduct of policymaking in both of these case studies, though it cannot be said that these policies would not have been implemented without these entrepreneurs. Their contribution is made not in agenda-setting but in the alternative selection and implementation phases.

## Poor Fit with Westminster Jurisdictions

Some findings undermine the utility of Kingdon's MS Framework for majoritarian, unitary Westminster systems, as they do not seem to conform to his predictions and therefore reduce confidence in the generalisability of his theory to these systems. Critics of Kingdon's MS Framework emphasise their concerns about the serendipitous elements of the framework and its lack of attention to collective approaches of individuals coming together to achieve a shared end, its US-centricity, the dependence in the theory upon opportunistic policy entrepreneurs as policy enablers to the exclusion of institutional or structural drivers or constraints upon policy change and its lack of recognition of the importance of historical antecedents. The case studies lend evidence to support this wide-ranging critique. In particular, many elements of Mucciaroni's critique, as they relate to the under-theorising of institutional factors (Mucciaroni 1992), are upheld.

Both case studies show non-serendipitous planned, top-down policymaking: each government was able to plan to introduce its preferred type of pay-for-performance policy (and its overarching reforms of health services) in the way and speed it preferred, taking careful account of the institutional arrangements in each jurisdiction. This offers support to the consensus in the literature, that policymaking has characteristics of greater autonomy in majoritarian unitary Westminster political systems, at least at the agenda-setting stage. The features of these political systems facilitate the management of top-down policymaking processes, which usually commence within political parties prior to an election and are implemented by an apolitical and experienced civil service immediately afterwards. Aberbach and Christensen have utilised the MS Framework to describe such a process in New Zealand in 1984 when dramatic public sector reform occurred. "The main vehicle of change was the Labour Party.... [The] strategy had a high probability of success in New Zealand's political-administrative system, dominated by an elective dictatorship" (Aberbach 2001, p. 419). Incoming governments can make major changes, at least initially, in the face of opposition from some interest groups. The particular risks faced by policymakers in Westminster jurisdictions are the difficulties in managing the implementation stage of policymaking and the risk that policies will be often overturned at the next change of administration.

## IDENTIFYING OTHER DRIVERS OF POLICY VARIATION AND CHANGE

The two processes of policymaking in these jurisdictions conform only partly with Kingdon's MS Framework. The particular features of these processes which seem to explain the nature of policy change in each case and the variation between the two cases are best captured in a mix of institutional and rational choice approaches to what happened and why. To isolate these, the key differences revealed in the two case studies are now set out.

### *Opportunity for Bargaining and Negotiation*

The most important aspect in which the two episodes of policymaking differ is the use of formal bargaining and negotiation processes in England and their absence in New Zealand. Because this bargaining approach encouraged the development of a larger scheme and achieved higher levels of engagement from general practitioners, it is also responsible for the difference in health outcomes attributable to the schemes in each case study.

### *England*
Bargaining processes used in England are evident in several key aspects of the policy design: the setting out of the initial principle that more pay would be conditional upon performance; the bargaining over the scheme itself including types of domains, health actions suitable to be included,

the nature of the indicators, the targets themselves and features of thresholds and exemptions within the scheme, and on the share of income dependent on performance. Many other aspects of the contract negotiation highlight the way participants faced choices in a context of explicit bargaining. This is perhaps axiomatic given that the process by which terms and conditions of work for general practitioners in England are set is through collective bargaining. Many efforts were made to ensure that principle-based bargaining occurred.

The fact that the QOF was part of the pay negotiation for general practices was a factor in its size and the speed of its implementation and comprehensiveness of take-up. The BMA and its members were impatient for an improvement in their terms and conditions of work and ready to concede increased oversight of the quality of their clinical practice to achieve a substantial lift in pay. This agreement was achieved through regular reporting back to the membership and formal processes of stage-by-stage voting, allowing members to participate directly in decisions about these new terms and conditions. General practitioners as members of the BMA approved the scheme by a majority vote and were well prepared for change arising from the settlement and thus for the implementation of the QOF itself.

The greater-than-expected cost of the new General Medical Services contract, as well as its speedy implementation, is a by-product of the strong incentives and drivers within the pay negotiation process at the heart of the new contract. Some fierce interest-based bargaining is certainly uncovered in the English case study evidence despite the attempts to minimise it through principle-based bargaining. This drove the generous out-of-hours settlement which, when the reduction of weekend surgery hours was apparent, had immediate negative repercussions for politicians. Within the QOF negotiation there was also some positional bargaining on the targets' degree of challenge, with one side wanting these to be "for work already being done" and the other wanting "to make it stretchy"; but comments such as it "felt like a practice meeting," which is a consensus-based process, were most common.

*New Zealand*

In New Zealand there was no existing institutional framework for the interests of general practitioners in this process of policy change to be formally bargained for or negotiated through a nationally representative forum. General practitioners closely associated with IPAs felt that this was, in the end, a zero-sum game of winners and losers which was seen by some participants as a "state-directed program." This conforms with Zahariadis' description of competitive networks which "appease certain critics ... and ... blatantly disregard the grievances of others" (Zahariadis 1995, p. 81). This approach resulted in disengagement and some bitterness about the process felt by some leaders of general practice and a reluctance to champion the scheme among their peers. It also reinforced the lack of a willingness by some general practice leaders to champion a project to develop a national database of practice performance in New Zealand, whereas this need was supported in England. If a database had been developed in New Zealand, it might have extended the range of indicators and therefore the value of the scheme to general practices and sped up processes of feedback to general practitioners themselves about their practice. In New Zealand the lack of timely feedback about performance exacerbated the low levels of engagement in its implementation. This contributed to the lower and slower levels of achievement of attributable health outcome gains (although the scheme was deliberately designed to be small and incremental because of caution about the mechanism of pay-for-performance).

It is impossible to know whether, in New Zealand, a mechanism for bargaining might have enabled resolution of the arguments over clinical leadership of the process and adequate access to patient treatment data. However, these issues were resolved in England.

### What Theories Best Explain This Evidence?

The major differences in the two case studies arise from institutional differences. Although the overarching governing structures are similar, differences in the systems for resourcing and remuneration of general practice services created a unique combination of institutional, rational choice and network drivers in each country which affected each policymaking process and the power of each state to strengthen its influence over providers of these services.

In England these include the mechanism of the General Medical Services contract and also the relationship between the BMA (the association representing the interests of general practitioners) and the state. Both of these features enabled the state to increase its leverage over the individual general practitioner's clinical behaviour by negotiating a conditional pay settlement. In this institutional framework bargaining was a rule of the game and general practitioners could negotiate a reduction in autonomy for a more valued improvement in their terms and conditions of work. They had little choice but to engage with the contract negotiation process if they wished to influence their terms and conditions of pay. They had to implement the pay-for-performance scheme if they wished to increase their income.

In New Zealand the state was able to implement a new contractual relationship with general practice, introduce patient registers and a new governance framework of PHOs. But it still had relatively little leverage over the individual general practitioner's behaviour. This institutional framework offered no opportunity for bargaining between the state and the profession. General practitioners did not have to implement the pay-for-performance scheme if they wished to increase their income, especially since the scheme was dependent upon PHOs and practices locally negotiating terms for general practitioners which did not always provide for rewards to be paid directly to practices. Where this was the case there was less incentive for practices to implement the pay-for-performance scheme.

New Zealand had very few existing central quality guidelines to build on and it was difficult to obtain clinical agreement on suitable targets for the pay-for-performance scheme. Because New Zealand policymakers were sceptical about pay-for-performance and individual general practitioners did not need pay-for-performance to increase their income, the incentives for both parties were against the design of a large scheme.

Theories which combine institutional and rational actor approaches (Tuohy 1999, 2012; Crouch 2005) emphasise the role of individual actors in health policymaking. In the case studies for this research, actors from general practice are seen to be taking an innovative approach to designing new governance mechanisms for clinical practice, enabling funders and patient representatives to be included in debates over clinical practice which were usually conducted within the profession. These actors undoubtedly facilitated the policymaking process. There are significant differences in the general practice networks in each country. In general terms the English network can be described as having greater unity, fewer and stronger structural forms, a more consensual mode that facilitated communication between members, higher capacity and more restricted access to membership and guaranteed access to decision-makers. Such networks, in Zahariadis' terms, have a trajectory of incremental and emergent development of a policy idea or "rapid propulsion to salience of a persistently softened idea" (Zahariadis 1995, p. 73). The New Zealand network is at the other end of the continuum with considerable heterogeneity, multiple, loosely organised structures, more competitive modes which retarded communication between members, lower administrative capacity and less restricted access to membership, and had patchy access to decision-makers. In such networks a more "quantum" pattern of initial change may occur but then a more gradualist pathway towards unified adoption will be observed. Each country displays a different trajectory. The English sub-system displays "rapid propulsion" to pay-for-performance after a period of "softening up" in the fund-holding era. The New Zealand sub-system displays initial quantum change in take-up of local budget management contracts but then gradual progress towards adoption of a national pay-for-performance scheme.

The history of relationships between the government and the interest groups also exerted influence and provided important context for the policymaking differently in each case. In England the "politics of the double bed" had been reinstated by the Labour government in 1997. In such a working relationship the "logic of exchange stresses common interests and a search for unanimity" (Zahariadis 1995, p. 74). In New Zealand the relationship is identified as "a fundamentally conflicted one" (Croxson 2009, p. 33) in the evaluation of the primary health-care reforms, which also identified that the government "had no formal contractual means for meeting some of its objectives [and that] trust is a key informal arrangement in this type of environment—so if it is missing … a vital component of the informal institutional arrangements is also missing" (Croxson 2009, p. 36).

Two drivers of change and variation had relatively similar effects in both case studies:

**Socio-economic factors:** Both countries were in a period of strong economic growth and politicians had resolved to invest more resources in health care. So both schemes could be funded from new appropriations rather than making retention of existing levels of funding conditional upon new quality standards. This is undoubtedly an important feature which encouraged the design of both schemes. It can be assumed that the process of scheme design would have been more challenging and controversial in both countries if they had sought to make the use of existing income for general practitioners conditional upon new quality standards.

However, the evidence shows that policymakers in both countries were driven by concerns about significant socio-economic risks and pressures in the future if chronic health conditions were not better managed through population-based approaches to health outcomes.

**Ideas:** Consistent with the view that "purchasing systems are still very much path dependent—that is today's choices are limited by what has gone before" (Figueras 2005, p. 45), the content of the new policy in each case study draws heavily on existing models or familiar systems and that these in turn were based on New Public Management ideas.

The evidence shows that the ministers in both jurisdictions supported the idea of pay-for-performance within general practice and championed its use. Civil servants and general practitioners in both jurisdictions had mixed views, some believing strongly in its merits and seeking actively to implement it and others concerned about its risks or morally opposed to it. Participants reported that this mixture of attitudes to the idea of pay-for-performance was widespread. There was a greater degree of scepticism for the idea reflected in the New Zealand policy, policymakers choosing an incremental approach deliberately to minimise risk.

Together with the similar existing and predicted socio-economic environment shared by the two countries, the idea of pay-for-performance is a factor which, broadly speaking, affects both case studies equally. The evidence also illustrates the tenacity of politically partisan ideological preferences over time. In New Zealand these were very explicit and included the championing by the incoming Labour government of primary health-care team approaches over general practice leadership approaches and community-governed services over clinically led services. Starke has assessed the 25-year period of health reform in New Zealand as being driven by multi-causal factors but dominated by the tendency, when a moment of political opportunity presents itself, to turn to ideas already in the primeval policy soup but importantly, those that accord closely with partisan or party ideology (Starke 2010). In New Zealand's case this results in a pattern of reform and counter-reform in health policy. The establishment, abolition and re-instatement of regional health boards, initiated by successive governments, is a good example of this pattern. This pattern of reform and counter-reform is made more vivid by the shorter electoral term for administrations in New Zealand (three years as opposed to five years in England).

## IMPLICATIONS FOR KINGDON'S MS FRAMEWORK

It is not possible to make sense of these studies without taking into account the structural, institutional, rational choice and network factors which impinged so strongly on both policymaking processes. The effect of structural and institutional factors has been pervasive and dominant in these studies of policy change. The explanatory power of Kingdon's multi-theoretic approach, as enhanced by Zahariadis, is much improved but does not yet encourage sufficient consideration of these factors, particularly structural and institutional ones. It emphasises chance and individual actors as policy entrepreneurs in agenda-setting and these factors did not ultimately drive change or explain variation in these two policy-making episodes. The MS Framework also focuses upon single events of policy agenda-setting and adoption and their outputs, rather than seeing policymaking processes in a longitudinal context, which is especially important in Westminster systems where policies can be short-lived or long-lived depending upon policymakers' choice of process. Neither does the MS Framework consider policy outcomes, in this way neglecting opportunities to observe policy evolution over time.

Taken together, these shortcomings under-theorise aspects of the policy change and variation observed in the case studies and do not accurately predict the circumstances under which purposeful and orderly policymaking can occur or how policymaking occurs in settings of goal and policy clarity.

## ENHANCING THE MS FRAMEWORK

Jones suggests that there is a need to develop and adapt key concepts within the MS Framework to enhance its explanatory nuances and to explore how well it competes with or complements other policy approaches (Jones 2015, p. 31). A key concept of the MS Framework is that non-incremental change arises in contexts of ambiguity, fluidity of participation and nuclear technology. A major finding from this research is that this is not always the case, especially in more orderly jurisdictions such as the United Kingdom and New Zealand. Non-incremental change can be planned for and implemented in an orderly way. Softening this central assumption of the MS Framework is an important step towards increasing its relevance for such jurisdictions.

With respect to its five key elements, Spohr, Béland and Zohlnhöfer, Herweg and Rüb have earlier been credited with research leading to the integration of MS Framework and historical institutionalist perspectives (Béland 2005; Zohlnhöfer 2016a, b). The studies described in this book have shown that institutional, rational actor and interest group or network approaches are all necessary to explain policymaking and to manage it more effectively in these jurisdictions. If the elements of Kingdon's MS

Framework as set out by Zahariadis were adapted to further integrate institutional concepts, this would increase its utility, especially for Westminster jurisdictions and for future policymaking generally. These enhancements are proposed as sub-elements capturing network and institutional variables to be added to Zahariadis' model.

The **institutional context,** including national-level political institutions but also forms of ownership and governance of public services (in particular the form pertaining to the system or sub-system related to the policymaking) is a key factor in policymaking. If consideration of this is encouraged within the **Politics** Stream, it would enable an assessment of the degree of autonomy the state, through its elected representatives, has to develop policy. This would not only enable options such as bargaining approaches to be assessed for feasibility in the policymaking process, but also enable consideration of which types of entrepreneur in which institutional positions may best be able to facilitate policymaking. More broadly it would invite questions about whether party ideology is important in agenda-setting. If so it will elevate consideration by policymakers of windows of opportunity arising from administrative turnover. In such an environment, greater consideration would be given to doctrinally driven policy ideas arising through political parties. This change would strengthen the relevance of the theory to a wider range of jurisdictions. It is suggested that this is added as a sub-element to the Politics Stream. Schlager also recommends that Kingdon's MS Framework be amended to incorporate institutional structure within the Politics Stream (Schlager 2007, p. 306).

This research has found that **institutional entrepreneurs** were important to the policymaking process, mandated by policymakers or decision-makers and often focusing their efforts on changing institutional frameworks to facilitate policy change as well as advocating for particular policies. This research makes the particular case to include institutional entrepreneurs in the **Entrepreneurs** Stream. Recommendations to recognise the role of "political entrepreneurs" flow from the work of Zohlnhöfer (2016b).

**Antecedent policies** or the policymaking history are an important feature of the two case studies and the literature suggests they are likely to be so in other policymaking situations. Kingdon acknowledges their importance. The presence or absence of antecedent policies as a sub-element of the **Policy** Stream is suggested as an enhancement to the model. In addition, consideration of its **outcome** is a missing element in Kingdon's policymaking framework as elaborated by Zahariadis. While the policy output is a focus in Zahariadis' model, it is incomplete without consideration of the policy outcome. Analysis of the outcome of a policymaking process would assist successive policymakers to make judgments about the costs and benefits of different approaches. It would inform subsequent cycles of policymaking, of which there may be many, repeated over many decades, as this case study has shown. Outcomes will not be known and understood at the time of policymaking but the desired outcome should be documented and achievements measured to provide a full picture of the policy-making process. There is a strong case for inclusion of a new element in the model—that of **policy outcome**—which would enhance or extend Kingdon's MS Framework for policy analysis. These proposed revisions to elements and sub-elements reflect the key institutional factors which are under-represented in the model.

## Summing Up: Research Findings and Looking Forward

This research has studied the policymaking process in two national settings using a novel synthesised analytical framework which tests the multi-theoretic MS Framework against five other single-driver theories of policy change and variation. The evolution of the MS Framework in recent years is acknowledged. However the findings of this research have led to recommendations for further enhancing the MS Framework to make it more useful in Westminster majoritarian unitary jurisdictions.

The research has also explored pay-for-performance health policymaking in two countries in 2001 when such schemes in national health systems were relatively untried. Over time, much new research about pay-for-performance has been completed and has drawn upon the experience of the QOF development in England. The research question today is not whether to use pay-for-performance but how best to incorporate it in financing arrangements for general practice services (Roland 2014), bearing in mind Saltman's warning that "the experience of one country with payment systems and financial incentives cannot easily be reproduced in another country—even if there is a high degree of cultural and institutional similarities" (Saltman 2005, p. 195). Given the passage of time there can also be an assessment of whether improved population-based health outcomes have been achieved by the initiatives in both countries.

As a further contribution from this research, some next steps are proposed for consideration by policymakers in New Zealand to achieve improved population-based health outcomes through primary health-care services. Policymakers could consider two difference scenarios for future policy development: incremental or non-incremental.

**Incremental style:** This would support the evolution of general practice institutional forms and interest group structures towards more collaborative types of political exchange over time. Four steps are recommended for consideration. First, in the case of New Zealand, this might include building on the achievements described in this research and introducing a stronger institutional context for building trust and collaboration within this sub-system such as mandating a single national representative body for general practice, perhaps consisting of a forum of representatives from the various segments of the general practice professional community. Such a body would have unrestricted access to government decision-makers regarding policymaking which affected general practice, utilising principle-based bargaining and negotiation processes. This could be expected to lead to slowly building greater mutual trust between general practitioners and the representative body and between that body and the state through repeated instances of consensus-based policymaking seen to balance the interest of both parties.

Secondly, New Zealand needs to support the enhancement of improved policy community resources for primary health care (including general practice) to inform policy ideas and develop information and knowledge infrastructure based on evidence. This could include investment of adequate resources to build a comprehensive shared database for primary care service delivery on the model of the QMAS and rapid development of an evidence base, shared national service frameworks and quality standards and targets on the model of the domains developed within the QOF.

Negotiating greater alignment between interest groups and policy specialists and the two major political parties on key aspects of population-based health policy would be another important step. A bi-partisan agreement to support the key elements of agreed infrastructure-building steps over a ten-year period, avoiding the regular cycle of policy windows at election time which can bring policy reversals, could be a first step towards achieving longer periods of time for policy changes to embed.

Finally, extending the engagement with an international policy community, particularly of countries with similar governing systems, to support these developments would be important. A more extensive network and community of practice in this field of knowledge, which draws on other policy community resources, would enhance the resources of the New Zealand policy community for general practice and primary care policymaking.

**Non-incremental style:** New Zealand policymakers could commence further reforms of the ownership and governance frameworks for general practice services by negotiating with the profession to implement major structural change (such as a single-payer financing arrangement in general practice). Costly in terms of meeting the full and reasonable costs of general practice services through public funding, a business case for such investment would need to be based on potential improvements in metrics such as reductions in the health-care costs of chronic conditions and reduction in ambulatory-sensitive admissions which would arise from improved access to high-quality general practice services. Introduction of a broader-based pay-for-performance scheme in England has demonstrated the potential to deliver savings arising from anticipated reductions in ambulatory-sensitive admissions to more costly hospital-based care.

### Other Comparative Cases

Australia is a federal Westminster-style adversarial political system, having a universal comprehensive government-sponsored medical care insurance scheme (Medicare) that guarantees citizens free treatment in public hospitals and subsidised access to primary care (Nicholson 2012). Australia, facing problems of poor coordination between state and federal systems, launched a national primary health-care strategy in 2010. It, too, implemented a pay-for-performance scheme in 2001, the Practice Incentives Program (PIP), which has expanded from 3 to 11 domains, incentivising good quality in key chronic disease domains such as diabetes, asthma, and indigenous and aged health-care domains. The scheme has the active involvement of doctors, rewards individual practices and groups, and rates well in Eijkenaar's Appropriate Design measures for pay-for-performance schemes (Eijkenaar 2013). There is mixed evidence about its effectiveness in improving quality over time, with an evaluation of gains in diabetes management in 2009 finding the probability of HbA1c testing by 20 percentage points with the strongest effect on patients from indigenous backgrounds (more than 35 percentage points) (Scott 2009), but a subsequent study by Greene (2013) disputing the strength of the scheme impact and suggesting refinements to improve its attraction to general practitioners. Close to home for New Zealand policymakers, Australia offers a comparative example of thorough-going but incremental change in the relationship between general practitioners and the state, evolving towards shared goals and mutually trusting working relationships.

Canada offers an example of a jurisdiction which successfully achieved a non-incremental policy change in general practice governance when it introduced a single-payer framework late in the development of its health system. A Westminster-style adversarial political system with a federal structure, its universal comprehensive government-sponsored medical care insurance scheme was legislated for in 1966 and finally fully implemented in 1971 (Tuohy 1999, pp. 93–95). With respect to both constitutional structure and timing, Canada does not offer so close a match to the New Zealand case study as England does, except for a key feature. During implementation, and in a replay of the accommodation reached between the state and medical profession in New Zealand in 1948, several Canadian provinces allowed doctors to "extra-bill" patients in exchange for accepting the state as the sole funder of medical and hospital services. Concern about financial barriers to care arose during the 1980s in Canada as it did in New Zealand. The practice of extra-billing was nevertheless outlawed in 1984 in Canada as a result of a campaign by a Liberal government with declining popularity, seeking the "product differentiation" typical in an adversarial electoral system. This campaign promise to end extra-billing was seized upon and joined by the opposition party for its own electoral advantage and implemented. After some bitter opposition, the profession has preserved considerable clinical autonomy but surrendered some entrepreneurial autonomy to the state in its role of funder.

A non-incremental change of this nature in New Zealand would require bi-partisan political support based on public interest principles. It may take many years to design and implement constructively, drawing on the experience and advice of governments and general practice organisations in England (and Scotland) and Canada to give a complete picture of the costs and benefits for both parties to the arrangements. It would also be an appropriate environment for the activities of institutional entrepreneurs to be recruited by the state. New institutional arrangements would be the key output of such policymaking. New collaborative working relationships between the state and general practitioners and improved population health would be the sought-after outcomes.

In both scenarios, skilful engagement by the state of entrepreneurial actors with a specific brief to pursue continuing institutional innovation is likely to be a facilitating factor in the speed, nature and extent of policy-making change.

## NOTES

1. http://www.health.govt.nz/nz-health-statistics/health-statistics-and-data-sets/primary-care-data-and-stats

## REFERENCES

Aberbach, J. D., & Christensen, T. (2001). Radical Reform in New Zealand: Crisis, Windows of Opportunity, and Rational Actors. *Public Administration, 79*(2), 403–422.

Béland, D. (2005). Ideas and Social Policy: An Institutional Perspective. *Social Policy and Administration, 39*(1), 1–18.

Comptroller and Auditor General. (2008). *NHS Pay Modernisation: New Contracts for General Practice Services in England*. London: National Audit Office.

Comptroller and Auditor General. (2010). *Tackling Inequalities in Life Expectancy in Areas with the Worst Health and Deprivation*. London: National Audit Office.

Cranleigh Health. (2012). *PHO Performance Programme Evaluation*. Auckland: Cranleigh Health.

Crouch, C. (2005). *Capitalist Diversity and Change*. Oxford: Oxford University Press.

Croxson, B., Smith, J., & Cumming, J. (2009). *Patient Fees as a Metaphor for So Much More in New Zealand's Primary Health Care System*. Wellington: Health Services Research Centre, Victoria University of Wellington.

Dixon, A., Khachatryan, A., Wallace, A., Peckham, S., Boyce, T., & Gillam, S. (2010). *The Quality and Outcomes Framework (QOF): Does It Reduce Health Inequalities?* Final Report. London: National Institute for Health Research.

Eijkenaar, F., Emmert, M., Scheppach, M., & Schoffski, O. (2013). Effects of Pay for Performance in Health Care: A Systematic Review of Systematic Reviews. *Health Policy, 110*, 115–130.

Figueras, J., Robinson, R., & Jajubowski, E. (2005). *Purchasing to Improve Health Systems Performance*. Copenhagen: World Health Organisation.

Greene, J. (2013). An Examination of Pay-for-performance in General Practice in Australia. *Health Services Research, 48*(4), 1415–1418.

John, P. (1998). *Analysing Public Policy*. London: Cassell.

Jones, M., Peterson, H., Pierce, J., Herweg, N., Bernal, A., Raney, H. L., et al. (2015). A River Runs Through It: A Multiple Streams Meta-review. *Policy Studies Journal, 44*(1), 13–36.

McDonald, R., Cheraghi-Sohi, S., Tickle, M., Roland, M., Doran, T., Campbell, S., et al. (2010). The *Impact of Incentives on the Behaviour and Performance of Primary Care Professionals.* Report for the National Institute for Health Research Service Delivery and Organisation Programme Manchester, National Institute for Health Research Service Delivery and Organisation Programme.

Ministry of Health. (2014). *Integrated Performance and Incentive Framework Expert Advisory Group.* Final Report. Health. Wellington: Ministry of Health.

Mucciaroni, G. (1992). The Garbage Can Model & the Study of Policy Making: A Critique. *Polity, 24*(3), 459–482.

Nicholson, C., Jackson, C., Marley, J., & Wells, R. (2012). The Australian Experiment: How Primary Care Organisations Supported the Evolution of a Primary Health Care System. *Journal of American Board of Family Medicine, 25*(Suppl), S18–S26.

PHO Performance Programme. (2010). *PHO Performance Programme Annual Report 1 July 2009–30 June 2010.* Wellington: District Health Boards New Zealand.

PHO Performance Programme. (2011). *PHO Performance Programme Annual Report 1 July 2010–30 June 2011.* Wellington: District Health Boards Shared Services.

Pollitt, C., Harrison, S., Dowswell, G., Bal, R., & Jerak-Zuiderent, S. (2008). *Performance Indicators: A Logic of Escalation?* European Group for Public Administration Conference. Rotterdam: Erasmus University.

Przeworski, A., & Teune, H. (1970). *The Logic of Comparative Social Inquiry.* New York: Wiley-Interscience.

Roland, M., & Campbell, S. (2014). Successes and Failures of Pay for Performance in the United Kingdom. *New England Journal of Medicine, 370*(20), 1944–1949.

Saltman, R., Rico, A., & Boerma, W. (2005). *Primary Care in the Drivers Seat?* Maidenhead: Open University Press.

Schlager, E. (2007). A Comparison of Frameworks, Theories, and Models of Policy Process. In P. Sabatier (Ed.), *Theories of the Policy Process.* Boulder: Westview Press.

Scott, A., Schurer, S., Jensen, P. H., & Sivey, P. (2009). The Effects of an Incentive Program on Quality of Care in Diabetes Management. *Health Economics, 18*(9), 1091–1108.

Starke, P. (2010). Why Institutions Are Not the Only Thing That Matters: Twenty-Five Years of Health Care Reform in New Zealand. *Journal of Health Politics, Policy and Law, 35*(4), 487–516.

Tenbensel, T., Mays, N., & Cumming, J. (2011). A Successful Mix of Hierarchy and Collaboration? Interpreting the 2001 Reform of the Governance of the New Zealand Public Health System. *Policy & Politics, 39*(2), 239–255.

Tuohy, C. H. (1999). *Accidental Logics.* Oxford: Oxford University Press.

Tuohy, C. H. (2012). *Institutional Entrepreneurs and the Politics of Redesigning the Welfare State: The Case of Health Care.* New Orleans, a paper to be presented at the annual meeting of the American Political Science Association, New Orleans, Louisiana.

Zahariadis, N. (1995). Ideas, Networks, and Policy Streams: Privatization in Britain and Germany. *Policy Studies Review, 14,* 71–98.

Zohlnhöfer, R., & Rüb, F. (Eds.) (2016a). *Decision-Making under Ambiguity and Time Constraints.* Colchester: ECPR Press.

Zohlnhöfer, R., Herweg, N., & Rüb, F. (2016b). Bringing Formal Political Institutions into the Multiple Streams Framework: An Analytical Proposal for Comparative Policy Analysis. *Journal of Comparative Policy Analysis, 18*(3), 243–256.

# CHAPTER 9

# Conclusion

**Abstract** A compelling case is made to adapt and improve the ability of Kingdon's Multiple Streams Framework to predict planned, purposeful and orderly non-incremental policymaking in majoritarian parliamentary jurisdictions. New Institutionalist, institutional rational choice and network literatures are used, in addition to Kingdon's Framework, to explain what happened in two case studies of pay-for-performance policymaking in general practice in England and New Zealand between 2001 and 2007. Rare rich descriptions of public policymaking in the general practice sub-systems of these two countries are delivered, offering many insights of both practical and theoretical assistance to those interested in the dynamics of policymaking.

**Keywords** Multiple Streams Framework • Pay-for-performance • Majoritarian parliamentary jurisdictions

Two Westminster states sought to increase incentives for improved population-based health outcomes in the general practice health sub-system. An opportunity presented by a quasi-natural experiment in these two countries has been utilised to explore these two case studies of the design of a pay-for-performance scheme, opening a window on "private negotiations between tight networks" (Marsh 2001, p. 196) and rare rich descriptions of

© The Author(s) 2018
V. Smith, *Bargaining Power*,
https://doi.org/10.1007/978-981-10-7602-2_9

public policymaking in both countries. The comparative approach considered the policy goal and policy instrument, timing, governing systems, type of health system, history of health sector reform and general practice subsystem institutional and network features in each country.

Key institutional enablers assisted England to engage general practitioners successfully in policymaking. This created a context for rational choice drivers to lead to policymaking which increased the influence of the state over general practice activities. While New Zealand has taken important steps towards achieving its policymaking goals, its general practice institutional features acted as constraints on pay-for-performance policymaking. These differences include the multiple forms of ownership and governance of general practice services, the systems for resourcing and remuneration, multiplicity of interest groups and low levels of integration of the policy community in the general practice sector in New Zealand. These differences, especially in the systems for resourcing and remuneration, reduced the power of politicians to achieve a significant shift in their influence over general practice services. This in turn affects the ability of the state to exercise effective stewardship over all the public investment in its health system. In New Zealand evidence shows that the degree of genuine engagement with a large segment of the general practice sector in the policymaking process was low. Without such engagement, the risk of lack of adoption of the policy and the delivery of its benefits by that section of general practitioners was high. With greater engagement, the opportunity to design a larger pay-for-performance scheme with greater influence on health inequalities might have been achieved. However, with the assistance of entrepreneurial actors, new forms of governance have been developed, which recombine successful mechanisms from adjacent areas, including IPAs and community-led primary health-care services, and Māori and Pacific institutional approaches to equity-based service delivery.

Both case studies show that non-incremental change in primary care health policy can be achieved by governments wanting to improve health outcomes for citizens and that general practitioners can be incentivised to take a population-based approach to their work. However, politicians need to carefully assess the scale, pace, and scope of such change in light of the institutional features of their general practice sub-system.

The utility of Kingdon's MS Framework in describing and explaining these two episodes of policymaking in Westminster jurisdictions is challenged by the case studies. The patterns of change found in the research run counter to those predicted in Kingdon's MS Framework for the conditions associated with non-incremental change. However, Kingdon's multi-theoretic approach is valuable in taking a systemic approach to the analysis of each policymaking episode, demonstrating the interactivity of streams, elements and sub-elements and acknowledging human agency. Kingdon's MS Framework captures the complexity of policymaking in the studies better than a single approach would have done. It confirms that his work has been helpfully enhanced by the work of Zahariadis, which has deconstructed elements of agenda-setting and alternative selection processes, setting these out in an analytical framework and extending it to reflect on network factors such as the effects of policy community integration on the type of policy change.

However, the MS Framework continues to underestimate the importance of structural and institutional features in policymaking in Westminster jurisdictions which permit more purposeful and orderly policymaking while still achieving non-incremental change. Enhancements to the MS Framework to heighten its consideration of structural and institutional factors are necessary. If outcomes of policymaking as well as outputs are considered in the Framework to show what has and has not worked, and why, it will deliver improved guidance for future policymaking.

Despite differences in the scope and effectiveness of the pay-for-performance policies in each jurisdiction, both states are shown to have held and exercised considerable powers to design and drive through wide-ranging health system reform in planned, top-down processes. They both sought to use non-confrontational methods of engagement with key interest groups where possible, in order to distinguish themselves from attempts of previous administrations to impose unwanted change.

How states can achieve major change to improve health outcomes for citizens is part of their challenge of health system stewardship. Both governments held high hopes on behalf of citizens for system-wide health reform when they came into office. The examination of these reform efforts provides greater understanding about what drove policy change and variation and may make it easier for future governments to fulfil their hopes for improved health outcomes for citizens.

## Reference

Marsh, D., Richards, D., & Smith, M. J. (2001). *Changing Patterns of Governance in the United Kingdom*. Basingstoke: Palgrave Macmillan.

# Appendix

## Methods

A comparative case study methodology in a most-similar-systems design (Yin 2009) was used to explore the policymaking process in two countries, based on purposeful selection. A key research question was "In what aspects and why did two similar episodes of policy formulation and implementation in two similar jurisdictions follow different processes and have different outcomes?" The unit of analysis was the process of policy design of the pay-for-performance component of primary health care policy changes. The focus was on the processes of agenda-setting and alternative selection leading to policy formulation and authoritative decision (Kingdon 2010). However, evidence from the ten-year period before and after the policymaking period and evaluations of the schemes was also considered.

A qualitative methodology was adopted, utilising documentary analysis and seeking semi-structured interviews with 26 proximate decision-makers, leaders, and participants who were directly engaged in the design of the two pay-for-performance systems. Ethics approval was gained from the relevant bodies in both England and New Zealand to interview people identified by their managing organisations as negotiating the terms and conditions of the pay-for-performance schemes. They were invited to participate in a one-hour interview and asked about their role in the process of policy design and/or implementation, their perception of the dynamics in the process of design, what their expectations about the process had been and to what extent these were realised.

© The Author(s) 2018
V. Smith, *Bargaining Power*,
https://doi.org/10.1007/978-981-10-7602-2

Interviews were transcribed immediately, and the process of interviewing them was continued until no new data was appearing and saturation was achieved. Analysis of the transcribed interviews proceeded inductively, involving reading and re-reading the data and note-taking (rather than coding) of themes, looking for patterns in the data and the prevalence and strength of themes (Braun 2006). A comprehensive description was developed of the processes of policymaking from the point of view of each participant (who did what, when, how and why). This was cross-checked and corroborated against the data collected from other participants and from documentary evidence available to the researcher, such as government reports and media reports, to validate the causes, consequences and relationships which appeared in the data. Then tables setting out patterns of similarity and difference in descriptions of processes by role of participant (such as politician, doctor, civil servant) were developed and considered, in order to understand whether there was evidence of common role-based expression of interests or understandings. The data corpus was then written up as two case study narratives which described what happened, why and how this was perceived by different participants. These case studies were then re-submitted as summaries to all interviewees from each country case study for verification, cross examination and testing of trustworthiness of the analysis. These summaries included the data induced by the researcher though thematic analysis, as well as extensive descriptive material drawn directly from participants, in a process to seek validation of these conclusions. All participants responded and minor changes were made to the analysis following this process.

As part of each case study, structural and historical contexts were described and points of structural similarity between both countries noted, such as their political and health systems. Points of historical divergence, such as the relationship between state funders and general practitioners, were also noted. These cases were then compared using a cross-case synthesis technique (Yin 2009, p. 156) to develop a set of similarities and differences and apply Castles' attribution process (Castles 1991) to "locate some particular features in which otherwise very similar nations differ (so that) we are entitled to suggest it is attributable to one of the few other factors distinguishing them." In this analytical process, the dependent variable was the policy outcome and all other variables, including institutional, network-based, socio-economic, ideational and rational actor explanations were explored as independent variables. The research sought to establish the relationships between variables which could be identified from the analysis to explain the results. The utility of literatures on causes of policy change and variation, namely institutional, network-based, socio-economic, ideational and rational actor-based theories of policy change and variation, as set out by John (John 1998), and the utility of Kingdon's multi-theoretic Multiple Streams Framework (Kingdon 2010) was applied to each case.

## LIMITATIONS

Some limitations apply to this research. First, the research largely reflects the interpretation of events by elites, leaders and entrepreneurs who participated in the policymaking process rather than the views of general practitioners who were not active participants in the policymaking process. Second, the events described by participants had taken place at least seven years prior to the interviews for this research so inevitably the passage of time affected the recall of these events by participants. This also gives some time for reflection from a distance.

Some participants who contributed to setting the goals of the policymaking process declined to be interviewed for the case study of the Quality and Outcomes Framework, and I was unable to obtain access to documentary evidence relevant to that case study despite making repeated formal requests for it. I was also unable to obtain working papers for the Referred Services Expert Advisory Group in New Zealand. In both cases these additional documentary sources would have enabled more accurate tracing of the minuted decision-making processes in each policymaking episode.

Participants shared their understanding of the goals, objectives and conduct of the policymaking process as they interpreted and experienced them. My own judgments about the relative importance of the information I collected added a further interpretive layer. The corroborative processes which I undertook, in particular by offering the opportunity to all participants to read and comment upon the chapter which described the case study of policymaking in which they were participants were important safeguards against bias and partiality. This process was undertaken by the majority of participants and resulted in minor changes to the text in the description of both case studies.

# REFERENCES

Aberbach, J. D., & Christensen, T. (2001). Radical Reform in New Zealand: Crisis, Windows of Opportunity, and Rational Actors. *Public Administration, 79*(2), 403–422.

Audit Commission. (2011). *Paying GPs to Improve Quality*. London: Audit Commission.

Barnett, P., Malcolm, L., Wright, L., & Hendry, C. (2004). Professional Leadership and Organisational Change: Progress Towards Developing a Quality Culture in New Zealand's Health System. *The New Zealand Medical Journal, 117*, 1198.

Barnett, P., Tenbensel, T., Cumming, J., Clayden, C., Ashton, T., Pledger, M., et al. (2009). Implementing New Modes of Governance in the New Zealand Health System: An Empirical Study. *Health Policy, 93*, 118–127.

Béland, D. (2005). Ideas and Social Policy: An Institutional Perspective. *Social Policy and Administration, 39*(1), 1–18.

Belgrave, M. (1985). *"Medical Men" and "Lady Doctors": The Making of a New Zealand Profession 1867–1941*. PhD thesis, Victoria University of Wellington, New Zealand.

Belich, J. (1996). *Making Peoples*. Auckland: Allen Lane.

Belich, J. (2001). *Paradise Reforged*. Auckland: Allen Lane.

Blair, T. (2010). *A Journey*. London: Hutchinson.

Blank, R., & Burau, V. (2006). Setting Health Priorities Across Nations: More Convergence Than Divergence? *Journal of Public Health Policy, 27*(3), 265–281.

Bolitho, D. G. (1984). Some Financial and Medico-Political Aspects of the New Zealand Medical Profession's Reaction to the Introduction of Social Security. *New Zealand Journal of Health, 18*(1), 34–49.

© The Author(s) 2018
V. Smith, *Bargaining Power*,
https://doi.org/10.1007/978-981-10-7602-2

161

Boston, J., Martin, J., Pallot, J., & Walsh, P. (Eds.). (1991). *Reshaping the State.* Auckland: Oxford University Press.

Braun, V., & Clarke, V. (2006). Using Thematic Analysis in Psychology. *Qualitative Research in Psychology, 3,* 77–101.

British Medical Association. (2013). How We Work. Retrieved 19 May 2013. https://www.bma.org.uk/about-us/how-we-work

Brown, M. C., & Crampton, P. (1997). New Zealand Policy Strategies Concerning the Funding of General Practitioner Care. *Health Policy, 41,* 87–104.

Buhr, K. (2012). The Inclusion of Aviation in the EU Emissions Trading Scheme: Temporal Conditions for Institutional Entrepreneurship. *Organization Studies, 33*(11), 1565–1587.

Burau, V., & Blank, R. (2006). Comparing Health Policy: An Assessment of Typologies of Health Systems. *Journal of Comparative Policy Analysis, 8*(1), 63–76.

Campbell, A. (2012). *Power & Responsibility 1999–2001.* London: Arrow Books.

Campbell, S., Kontopantelis, E., Hannon, K., Burke, M., Barber, A., & Lester, H. (2011). Framework and Indicator Testing Protocol for Developing and Piloting Quality Indicators for the UK Quality and Outcomes Framework. *BMC Family Practice, 12,* 85.

Castles, F. G. (1991). *Australia Compared.* Sydney: Allen & Unwin.

Chaix-Coutourier, C., Durand-Zaleski, I., Jolly, D., & Durieux, P. (2000). Effects of Financial Incentives on Medical Practice: Results from a Systematic Review of the Literature and Methodological Issues. *International Journal for Quality in Health Care, 12*(2), 133–142.

Cohen, M., March, J., & Olsen, J. (1972). A Garbage Can Model of Organisational Choice. *American Science Quarterly, 17,* 1–25.

Comptroller and Auditor General. (2008). *NHS Pay Modernisation: New Contracts for General Practice Services in England.* London: National Audit Office.

Comptroller and Auditor General. (2010). *Tackling Inequalities in Life Expectancy in Areas with the Worst Health and Deprivation.* London: National Audit Office.

Crampton, P. (2000). Policies for General Practice. In P. Davis & T. Ashton (Eds.), *Health and Public Policy in New Zealand.* Auckland: Oxford University Press.

Crampton, P., Davis, P., Lay-Yee, R., Raymont, A., Forrest, C., & Starfield, B. (2004). Comparison of Private For-profit with Private Community-Governed Not-for-profit Primary Care Services in New Zealand. *Journal of Health Services Research & Policy, 9*(Suppl 2), 17–22.

Cranleigh Health. (2012). *PHO Performance Programme Evaluation.* Auckland: Cranleigh Health.

Crouch, C. (2005). *Capitalist Diversity and Change.* Oxford: Oxford University Press.

Croxson, B., Smith, J., & Cumming, J. (2009). *Patient Fees as a Metaphor for So Much More in New Zealand's Primary Health Care System.* Wellington: Health Services Research Centre, Victoria University of Wellington.

Cumming, J., & Mays, N. (2002). Reform and Counter Reform: How Sustainable Is New Zealand's Latest Health System Restructuring? *Journal of Health Services Research & Policy*, 7(Suppl 1), 46–55.

Cumming, J., & Mays, N. (2011). New Zealand's Primary Health Care Strategy: Early Effects of the New Financing and Payment System for General Practice and Future Challenges. *Health Economics, Policy and Law*, 6, 1–21.

Davis, P., & Ashton, T. (2000). *Health Policy and Public Policy in New Zealand*. Auckland: Oxford University Press.

Davis, P., Gribben, B., Lay-Yee, R., & Scott, A. (2002). How Much Variation in Clinical Activity Is There Between General Practitioners? A Multi-level Analysis of Decision-Making in Primary Care. *Journal of Health Services Research & Policy*, 7(4), 202–208.

Devlin, N., Maynard, A., & Mays, N. (2001). New Zealand's New Health Sector Reforms: Back to the Future? *BMJ*, 322, 1171–1174.

Dixon, A., Khachatryan, A., Wallace, A., Peckham, S., Boyce, T., & Gillam, S. (2010). *The Quality and Outcomes Framework (QOF): Does It Reduce Health Inequalities?* Final Report. London: National Institute for Health Research.

Doran, T., & Roland, M. (2010). Lessons from Major Initiatives to Improve Primary Care in the United Kingdom. *Health Affairs*, 29(5), 1023–1029.

Doran, T., Kontopantelis, E., Valderas, J., Campbell, S., Roland, M., Salisbury, C., et al. (2011). Effect of Financial Incentives on Incentivised and Non-incentivised Clinical Activities: Longitudinal Analysis of Data from the UK Quality and Outcomes Framework. *BMJ*, 342, d3590.

Doran, T., Kontopantelis, E., Fullwood, C., Lester, H., Valderas, J., & Campbell, S. (2012). Exempting Dissenting Patients from Pay for Performance Schemes: Retrospective Analysis of Exception Reporting in the UK Quality and Outcomes Framework. *BMJ*, 344, e2405.

Eijkenaar, F., Emmert, M., Scheppach, M., & Schoffski, O. (2013). Effects of Pay for Performance in Health Care: A Systematic Review of Systematic Reviews. *Health Policy*, 110, 115–130.

Epstein, A., Thomas, H. L., & Hamel, M. B. (2004). Paying Physicians for High Quality Health Care. *New England Journal of Medicine*, 350(4), 406–409.

Figueras, J., Robinson, R., & Jajubowski, E. (2005). *Purchasing to Improve Health Systems Performance*. Copenhagen: World Health Organisation.

Finlayson, M. (2000). Policy Implementation and Modification. In P. Davis & T. Ashton (Eds.), *Health and Public Policy in New Zealand*. Auckland: Oxford University Press.

Flood, C. (2001). *Profiles of Six Health Care Systems*. Toronto: University of Toronto.

Fougere, G. (1993). Struggling for Control: The State and the Medical Profession in New Zealand. In F. W. Hafferty & J. B. McKinlay (Eds.), *The Changing Medical Profession*. Oxford: Oxford University Press.

Fougere, G. (2001). Transforming Health Sectors: New Logics of Organizing in the New Zeland Health System. *Social Science and Medicine, 52,* 1233–1242.

Gauld, R. (2003). One Country, Four Systems: Comparing Changing Helath Policies in New Zealand. *International Political Science Review, 24*(2), 199–218.

Gauld, R. (2009). *The New Health Policy.* Maidenhead: Open University Press.

Gauld, R., & Mays, N. (2006). Are New Zealand's New Primary Health Organsations Fit for Purpose? *BMJ, 333,* 1216–1218.

Greene, J. (2013). An Examination of Pay-for-performance in General Practice in Australia. *Health Services Research, 48*(4), 1415–1418.

Gribben, B., Coster, G., Pringle, M., & Simon, J. (2002). Quality of Care Indicators for Population-Based Primary Care in New Zealand. *New Zealand Medical Journal, 115*(1151), 163–166.

Ham, C. (2004). *Health Policy in Britain.* Basingstoke: Palgrave Macmillan.

Hannon, K., Lester, H., & Campbell, S. (2012). Patients' View of Pay for Performance in Primary Care: A Qualitative Study. *British Journal of General Practice, 62,* e322–e328.

Hanson, E. (1980). *The Politics of Social Security.* Wellington: Auckland University Press.

Hay, I. (1989). *The Caring Commodity.* Wellington: Oxford University Press.

Hefford, M., Crampton, P., & Foley, J. (2005). Reducing Health Disparities Through Primary Care Reform: The New Zealand Experiment. *Health Policy, 72,* 9–23.

John, P. (1998). *Analysing Public Policy.* London: Cassell.

Jones, M., Peterson, H., Pierce, J., Herweg, N., Bernal, A., Raney, H. L., et al. (2015). A River Runs Through It: A Multiple Streams Meta-review. *Policy Studies Journal, 44*(1), 13–36.

King, A. (2000). *The New Zealand Health Strategy.* Wellington: Ministry of Health.

King, A. (2001). *The Primary Health Care Strategy.* Wellington: Ministry of Health.

King, M. (2003). *The Penguin History of New Zealand.* Auckland: Penguin Books.

Kingdon, J. W. (2010). *Agendas, Alternatives, and Public Policies, Update Edition, with an Epilogue on Health Care.* London: Longmans.

Klein, R. (1990). The State and the Profession: The Politics of the Double Bed. *BMJ, 301,* 700–702.

Klein, R. (2006). *The New Politics of the NHS.* Abingdon: Radcliffe Publishing.

Kontopantelis, E., Springate, D., Reeves, D., Ashroft, D., Valdeas, J., & Doran, T. (2014). Withdrawing Performance Indicators: Retrospective Analysis of General Practice Performance under UK Quality and Outcomes Framework. *BMJ, 348,* g330.

Kusi-Ampofo, O., Church, J., Conteh, C., & Heinmiller, B. T. (2015). Resistance and Change: A Multiple Streams Approach to Understanding Health Policymaking in Ghana. *Journal of Health Politics Policy and Law, 40*(1), 195–219.

Laugesen, M. (2000). The Institutional Context. In P. Davis & T. Ashton (Eds.), *Health and Public Policy in New Zealand.* Auckland: Oxford University Press.

Laugesen, M., & Banducci, S. (2000). *Support for Health Care in the Welfare State: Australia, Britain, Canada, New Zealand and the United States.* Western Political Science Association Annual Meeting, San Jose, CA.

Lovell-Smith, J. B. (1966). *The New Zealand Doctor and the Welfare State.* Auckland: Blackwood and Janet Paul.

Malcolm, L. (2004). *Peer Review of Referred Services Management Documents.* M. o. Health. Wellington: Aotearoa Health.

Malcolm, L., & Mays, N. (1999a). New Zealand's Independent Practitioner Associations: A Working Model of Clinical Governance in Primary Care? *BMJ, 319,* 1340–1342.

Malcolm, L., Wright, L., Seers, M., & Guthrie, J. (1999b). An Evaluation of Pharmaceutical Management and Budget Holding in Pegasus Medical Group. *The New Zealand Medical Journal, 112,* 162–164.

Malcolm, L., Wright, L., & Barnett, P. (2000). Emerging Clinical Governance: Developments in Independent Practitioner Associations in New Zealand. *New Zealand Medical Journal, 113,* 33–36.

Mandelson, P., & Liddle, R. (1996). *The Blair Revolution.* London: Faber and Faber Limited.

Marsh, D., & Rhodes, R. A. W. (1992). *Policy Networks in British Government.* Oxford: Clarendon Press.

Marsh, D., Richards, D., & Smith, M. J. (2001). *Changing Patterns of Governance in the United Kingdom.* Basingstoke: Palgrave Macmillan.

Martin Jenkins & Associates Ltd. (2008). *Evaluation of the PHO Performance Programme.* Wellington.

Mays, N., & Hand, K. (2000). *A Review of Options for Health and Disability Support Purchasing in New Zealand.* Wellington: The Treasury.

McDonald, R., Cheraghi-Sohi, S., Tickle, M., Roland, M., Doran, T., Campbell, S., et al. (2010). The *Impact of Incentives on the Behaviour and Performance of Primary Care Professionals.* Report for the National Institute for Health Research Service Delivery and Organisation Programme Manchester, National Institute for Health Research Service Delivery and Organisation Programme.

McNamara, P. (2006). Foreword: Payment Matters? The Next Chapter. *Medical Care Research Review, 63*(Suppl 1), 5S–10S.

Minister of Health. (2007). *The Primary Health Care Strategy—Monitoring Its Achievements 2007: Memo to the Cabinet Social Development Committee.* Wellington: Health.

Ministry of Health. (2005). *PHO Performance Management Programme*. M. o. Health.

Ministry of Health. (2014). *Integrated Performance and Incentive Framework Expert Advisory Group*. Final Report. Health. Wellington: Ministry of Health.

Mintrom, M., & Norman, P. (2009). Policy Entrepreneurship and Policy Change. *Policy Studies Journal, 37*(4), 649–667.

Mintrom, M., & Vergari, S. (1996). Advocacy Coalitions, Policy Entrepreneurs, and Policy Change. *Policy Studies Journal, 24*(3), 420–434.

Mucciaroni, G. (1992). The Garbage Can Model & the Study of Policy Making: A Critique. *Polity, 24*(3), 459–482.

Mulgan, R. (1995). Democratic Failure of a Single Party Government. *Australasian Political Studies Association, 30*, 82–97.

Nicholson, C., Jackson, C., Marley, J., & Wells, R. (2012). The Australian Experiment: How Primary Care Organisations Supported the Evolution of a Primary Health Care System. *Journal of American Board of Family Medicine, 25*(Suppl), S18–S26.

Nolte, E., & McKee, M. (2008). *Caring for People with Chronic Conditions*. Maidenhead: Open University Press.

NZLP. (1999). *Labour on Health*. Wellington: New Zealand Labour Party.

O'Malley, C. (2003). *A Reality Check: The Early Sector Response to the Primary Health Care Strategy*. Wellington: Wellington Independent Practitioners Association and Compass Health.

OECD. (1987). *Financing and Delivering Health Care: A Comparative Analysis of OECD Countries*. Paris: OECD.

OECD. (1994). *The Reform of Health Care Systems*. Paris: OECD.

OECD. (2004). *Towards High Performing Health Systems*. Paris: OECD.

Oliver, T. R., & Paul-Shaheen, P. (1997). Translating Ideas into Actions: Entrepreneurial Leadership in State Health Care Reforms. *Journal of Health Politics, Policy and Law, 2*(3), 721–788.

PHO Performance Programme. (2010). *PHO Performance Programme Annual Report 1 July 2009–30 June 2010*. Wellington: District Health Boards New Zealand.

PHO Performance Programme. (2011). *PHO Performance Programme Annual Report 1 July 2010–30 June 2011*. Wellington: District Health Boards Shared Services.

Pollitt, C., & Bouckaert, G. (2011). *Public Management Reform*. Oxford: Oxford University Press.

Pollitt, C., Harrison, S., Dowswell, G., Bal, R., & Jerak-Zuiderent, S. (2008). *Performance Indicators: A Logic of Escalation?* European Group for Public Administration Conference. Rotterdam: Erasmus University.

Pollitt, C., Harrison, S., Dowswell, G., Jerak-Zuiderent, S., & Bal, R. (2010). Performance Regimes in Health Care: Institutions, Critical Junctures and the Logic of Escalation in England and the Netherlands. *Evaluation, 16*(1), 13–29.

Przeworski, A., & Teune, H. (1970). *The Logic of Comparative Social Inquiry.* New York: Wiley-Interscience.

Referred Services Advisory Group. (2002). *Referred Services Management: Building Towards Equity, Quality and Better Health Outcomes.* Wellington: Ministry of Health.

Richards, D., & Smith, M. (2002). *Governance and Public Policy in the UK.* Oxford: Oxford University Press.

Roberts, N. C., & King, P. (1991). Policy Entrepreneurs: Their Activity Structure and Function in the Policy Process. *Journal of Public Administration Research and Theory, 1*(2), 147–175.

Roland, M., & Campbell, S. (2014). Successes and Failures of Pay for Performance in the United Kingdom. *New England Journal of Medicine, 370*(20), 1944–1949.

Rosenthal, M., Frank, R. G., Zhongie, L., & Epstein, A. M. (2005). Early Experience with Pay-for-performance. *JAMA, 294*(14), 1788–1793.

Sabatier, P. a. W. (Ed.). (2014). *Theories of the Policy Process.* New York: Westview Press.

Saltman, R., Rico, A., & Boerma, W. (2005). *Primary Care in the Drivers Seat?* Maidenhead: Open University Press.

Schlager, E. (2007). A Comparison of Frameworks, Theories, and Models of Policy Process. In P. Sabatier (Ed.), *Theories of the Policy Process.* Boulder: Westview Press.

Scott, A., Schurer, S., Jensen, P. H., & Sivey, P. (2009). The Effects of an Incentive Program on Quality of Care in Diabetes Management. *Health Economics, 18*(9), 1091–1108.

Scott, C. (2001). *Public and Private Roles in Health Care Systems.* Buckingham: Open University Press.

Secretary of State for Health. (2000). The NHS Plan. Health, The Stationery Office.

Seddon, M. E., Marshall, M. N., Campbell, S. M., & Roland, M. O. (2001). Systematic Review of Studies of Quality of Clinical Care in General Practice in the UK, Australia and New Zealand. *Quality and Safety in Health Care, 10,* 152–158.

Seldon, A. (2007). *Blair Unbound.* London: Pocket Books.

Shaw, R., & Eichbaum, C. (2008). *Public Policy in New Zealand.* Auckland: Pearson Education.

Smith, J., & Mays, N. (2007). Primary Care Organisations in New Zealand and England: Tipping the Balance of the Health System in Favour of Primary Care? *International Journal of Health Planning and Management, 22,* 3–19.

Smith, J., Mays, N., Ovenden, C., Cumming, J., McDonald, J., & Boston, J. (2010). *Managing Mixed Financing of Privately Owned Providers in the Public Interest*. Wellington: Institute of Policy Studies.

Spohr, F. (2016). Path-Departing Labour-Market Reforms in the United Kingdom and Sweden. In R. Zohlnhöfer & F. W. Rüb (Eds.), *Decision-Making under Ambiguity and Time Constraints* (pp. 251–269). Colchester: ECPR Press.

Spooner, A., Chapple, A., & Roland, M. (2000). The PRICCE Project, National Primary Care Research and Development Centre, University of Manchester.

Starke, P. (2010). Why Institutions Are Not the Only Thing That Matters: Twenty-Five Years of Health Care Reform in New Zealand. *Journal of Health Politics, Policy and Law, 35*(4), 487–516.

Steele, N., & Shekelle, P. (2016). After 12 Years, Where Next for QOF? *BMJ, 354*(i4103). https://doi.org/10.1136/bmj.i4103.

Steinmo, S., Thelen, K., & Longstreth, F. (1992). *Structuring Politics: Historical Institutionalism in Comparative Analysis*. Cambridge: Cambridge University Press.

Stevens, S. (2004). Reform Strategies for the English NHS. *Health Affairs, 23*(3), 37–44.

Strand, M., & Fosse, E. (2011). Tackling Health Inequalities in Norway: Applying Linear and Non-linear Models in the Policymaking Process. *Critical Public Health, 21*(3), 373–381.

Tenbensel, T. (2008). How Do Governments Steer Health Policy? A Comparison of Canadian and New Zealand Approaches to Cost Control and Primary Health Care Reform. *Journal of Comparative Policy Analysis: Research and Practice, 10*(4), 347–363.

Tenbensel, T., Mays, N., & Cumming, J. (2011). A Successful Mix of Hierarchy and Collaboration? Interpreting the 2001 Reform of the Governance of the New Zealand Public Health System. *Policy & Politics, 39*(2), 239–255.

Tuohy, C. H. (1999). *Accidental Logics*. Oxford: Oxford University Press.

Tuohy, C. H. (2010). *Paths of Progress in Healthcare Reform: The Scale and Pace of Change in Four Advanced Nations*. American Political Science Association Annual Meeting, Washington, DC.

Tuohy, C. H. (2012). *Institutional Entrepreneurs and the Politics of Redesigning the Welfare State: The Case of Health Care*. New Orleans, a paper to be presented at the annual meeting of the American Political Science Association, New Orleans, Louisiana.

Tuohy, C. H., Flood, C. M., & Stabile, M. (2004). How Does Private Finance Affect Health Care Systems? Marshalling the Evidence from OECD Nations. *Journal of Health Politics, Policy and Law, 29*(3), 359–396.

Walker, S., Mason, A., Claxton, K., Cookson, R., Fenwick, E., Fleetcroft, R., et al. (2010, May). Value for Money and the Quality and Outcomes Framework in Primary Care in the UK NHS. *British Journal of General Practice, 60*(574), e213–e220.

WHO. (2000). *The World Health Report 2000.* Geneva: World Health Organisation.

Wilkes, C., & Shirley, I. (1984). *In the Public Interest.* Auckland: Benton Ross.

Yin, R. K. (2009). *Case Study Research.* Thousand Oaks: Sage.

Zahariadis, N. (1995). Ideas, Networks, and Policy Streams: Privatization in Britain and Germany. *Policy Studies Review, 14,* 71–98.

Zahariadis, N. (2003). Ambiguity and Choice in European Public Policy. *Journal of European Public Policy, 15*(4), 514–530.

Zahariadis, N. (2007). The Multiple Streams Framework. In P. A. Sabatier (Ed.), *Theories of the Policy Process.* Boulder: Westview Press.

Zohlnhöfer, R., & Rüb, F. (Eds.) (2016a). *Decision-Making under Ambiguity and Time Constraints.* Colchester: ECPR Press.

Zohlnhöfer, R., Herweg, N., & Rüb, F. (2016b). Bringing Formal Political Institutions into the Multiple Streams Framework: An Analytical Proposal for Comparative Policy Analysis. *Journal of Comparative Policy Analysis, 18*(3), 243–256.

# Index[1]

**A**

Aberbach, J., 137

Access, 12–15, 63, 65, 115, 116, 126, 140, 141, 146, 155

Accountability, 27, 84
  of GPs, 1, 4, 126, 127, 130, 134
  in New Zealand, 76, 77, 103

Actors, 9–11, 67, 68, 73, 74, 126, 130, 135, 136
  endogenous, 67, 70, 118
  entrepreneurial, 116, 154 (*see also* Entrepreneurs)

Admissions, ambulatory-sensitive, 55, 106, 107, 128, 131, 147

Agenda-setting, 10, 11, 67, 112, 126, 135
  and MS Framework, 63, 70, 71, 143, 144

Alternative selection, *see* MS Framework (Multiple Streams Framework)

Ambiguity, 10, 18, 60, 67, 112, 118, 135

lack of, 60, 70, 135, 143

Antecedents, 70, 71, 122, 136

Autonomy, 3, 63, 136, 144
  clinical, 22, 46, 72, 73, 98, 139, 148
  professional, 35, 42, 64, 101, 136

**B**

Balance of interests, 12, 15, 114

Bargaining, 14, 15, 42, 47, 64, 65, 68, 72, 73, 132, 133, 137–139, 146
  *See also* negotiations

Barriers, 5, 26, 44–49, 96, 102, 120, 129, 148

Bassett, M., 98

Béland, D., 17, 143

Blair, Tony, 34, 35

British Medical Association (BMA), 22, 39, 54, 62, 64, 65, 73, 100, 101, 126, 134
  competing interest, 47
  contract, 44, 47, 48

[1] Note: Page numbers followed by "n" refer to notes

© The Author(s) 2018
V. Smith, *Bargaining Power*,
https://doi.org/10.1007/978-981-10-7602-2

British Medical Association (BMA)
   (*cont.*)
   General Practitioners' Committee,
      36, 37, 45
   and government, 41, 48, 60, 68
   negotiations, 44, 73
   NZ members, 23, 24
   QOF, 50, 51, 53, 138
   Quality Sub Group, 49, 68
   and state, 72, 139
   2001 election, 36, 61, 62
   *See also* Confederation team
Buhr, K., 18


**C**
Capitation, 25, 28, 29, 96, 117, 126
Care, primary health, 4, 5, 55, 63, 82,
      83, 133
   New Zealand, 26, 77–79, 121, 134,
      146, 147 (*see also* Primary
      Health Organisation (PHO);
      Primary Health Care Strategy
      (PHCS))
Case studies, 2, 17, 61–65, 69, 70, 73,
      116, 118, 121, 153, 154,
      157–159
   New Zealand, 73, 103
Castles, F. G., 158
Centralism (England), 35–36
Challenges, technical, 49–53, 92,
      102
Change, 27–29, 120
   non-incremental, 10, 17, 18, 60,
      71, 112, 135
   *See also* Policy
Chisholm, John, 36, 37, 40, 42, 45,
      47, 50, 52, 53
Choice, rational, 2, 73, 137, 154
Civil servants, 11, 12, 38, 52, 66, 71,
      112, 116, 118, 119, 126, 133
Clinicians, 39, 46, 83, 104, 117, 130
   *See also* General practitioners

Closing the Gaps, 97
Cohen, M., 10
College of General Practice (NZ), 89
Comparison, England & NZ schemes,
      21, 91, 104, 126–128
Confederation team, 36, 42, 43, 46,
      48, 49, 52, 60, 65, 67, 68
Consensus, 47, 91, 93, 114, 117
Contracts, 27–29, 34, 36
   New Zealand, 24, 78, 79, 85, 88,
      113, 114, 128, 141
Coupling, 12–14, 17, 18, 66, 116
Cranleigh Health, 106
Crouch, C., 18, 113, 117
Cumming, J., ix


**D**
Data, 5, 56, 93, 94, 102, 103, 105,
      106, 127, 158
   access to, 51, 103
   practice, 45, 50, 51, 102, 127
   *See also* Quality Management
      Advisory System (QMAS)
Databases, 44, 55, 87, 102, 103
   national, 87, 94, 115, 121, 130,
      139
   shared, 64, 146
   *See also* Information
Davis, P., 81
Decision style, 12, 14, 66, 116
Design, 2, 60, 64, 93, 101, 103, 105,
      120, 141
   and implementation, 60, 72, 73, 92,
      97, 106, 112
   Performance Plan (PP), 98, 102,
      106, 107, 117
   process, 41, 50, 69, 72, 73, 80, 95,
      130
   team, 65, 126
   *see also* Policy, design
District Health Boards (DHBs), 77,
      84, 88, 118, 121

Doran, T., 54
Drivers, 2, 64, 65, 70, 119, 120,
    125–128, 131, 132, 141
    rational choice, 73, 139, 154

E
Eijkenaar, F., 147
Election, 11, 13, 130
    England, 33, 36, 48, 60–63
    NZ, 23–25, 75, 76, 130
Enablers, 44–49, 96, 136, 154
Entrepreneurs, 16–19, 117, 118, 136,
    143
    institutional, vi, 68, 69, 113, 116,
        117, 144, 154
    policy, 11, 12, 14, 67, 68, 74, 112,
        116, 135

F
Farrar, Mike, 36, 41–44, 47, 50–53
Feasibility, technical, 11–13, 15, 63,
    64, 115, 121
Features, institutional and structural,
    71, 73, 119, 120, 126, 132, 154,
    155, 158
Feedback, 12, 61, 71, 84, 85, 95, 104,
    113, 131, 139
Fee-for-service, 25, 28, 29, 82, 90,
    96
Fees, 26, 28, 29, 39
Finlayson, M., 81, 120
Focusing events, 12, 61, 113
Fougere, G., 23
Framework, see MS Framework
    (Multiple Streams Framework);
    P&IF; Quality and Outcomes
    Framework (QOF)
Friendly Society, 25
Funders, state, 1, 27, 103, 158
Funding, 3, 28, 29, 84, 88, 96, 113,
    117, 129, 133, 141

New Zealand, 25–27, 76–79,
    83–85, 116, 130, 147;
    capitated, 84, 88, 96, 113, 117,
        126, 129
    for referred services, 86, 116

G
Garbage Can Model, 10
General Medical Services, 26
    contract, 34, 44, 60, 64, 66, 70,
        129, 138
General practitioners, see British
    Medical Association (BMA); GPs;
    Profession
Governance, 1, 18, 28, 73, 74, 112,
    122, 123, 154
    clinical, 78, 79, 84–87, 89, 92, 106,
        115
    in England, 134
    in New Zealand, 4, 73, 77, 95, 96,
        99, 116–120, 131, 140, 141,
        147, 148
Government, 3, 4, 28, 70, 73, 101,
    102, 127, 128, 132, 134
    change of, 12, 16, 117, 122
    England, 34, 40, 42, 43, 61, 65,
        129, 141
    and interest groups, 27, 82, 141
    New Zealand, 23–25, 75, 76,
        82–84, 87, 98, 121
GPs, 28, 29, 38, 48, 50, 51, 126, 127
    in England, 35
    in New Zealand, 87, 96, 125–128
Greene, J., 147

H
Health and Disability Services Act
    1993, 27
Health care, 4, 26, 35, 82, 131, 141
    preventive, 45, 76, 91, 117 (see also
        Primary health care)

Health outcomes, *see* Outcomes
History, 3, 4, 15, 103, 116, 126, 127,
    132, 134, 141, 144
    England, 21, 25–27, 47
    New Zealand, 23–28, 76, 81, 99,
        100, 122
    of policies, 63, 64, 69–72, 118,
        119, 122, 144
Hutton, John, 34–39, 41, 44–50


I
Idea, *see* Policy, idea
Ideology, 17, 62, 89, 114, 132, 142,
    144
    Party Ideology, 12, 14
Implementation (of schemes), 5, 11,
    43, 94, 95, 120–122, 157
    comparison, 127, 129, 130, 132
    in England, 35, 45, 51, 54, 55, 64,
        106, 139
    of indicators, 87, 88, 94
    in MS Framework, 11, 118
    in NZ, 81, 88, 99, 102
    PHCS, 113, 114, 116
    *See also* Design, and implementation
Incentives, 5, 6, 34, 46, 49, 50, 86,
    104, 105, 120, 140, 153
    financial, 5, 6, 46, 84, 91, 131,
        145
    insufficient, 55, 81
Independent Practitioners'
    Associations (IPAs), 28, 29,
    78–80, 94, 101, 102, 138
    and budgets, 92, 122
    and PHOs, 84, 90, 93, 98
Indicators, 41, 46, 49, 86–88, 91,
    127, 128, 130, 138, 139
    clinical, 38, 54, 88, 94, 106
Inequalities, 54, 82, 93, 117, 118
    health, 34, 44, 55, 77, 90, 97, 154
Inequities, 26, 39, 90, 96, 113

Information, 130
    systems, 80, 86, 105, 118, 121,
        129, 130
    technology, 15, 43, 54, 105
    *See also* Data; Databases
Institutional context, 12, 13, 66, 71,
    144, 146
Institutions, 2, 10, 16–18, 48, 119
    and MS Framework, 14–19
Integrated Performance and Incentive
    Framework, 130
Interaction, patterns of, 46–49, 99–102
Interest groups, 2, 11, 12, 46–49, 65,
    73, 82, 114, 141, 146, 158
    practitioners, 27, 82
Interests, 10, 65, 79, 92, 106, 138
    balance of, 12, 15, 114
    common, 141, 158
    competing, contending, 47, 60, 118
    different, 24, 47, 73, 89, 135
    funder, 46, 86, 98


J
John, P., 2, 10, 132
Jones, M., 143
Junior minister, *see* Hutton


K
King, Annette, 81, 82, 99, 100
    *See also* Minister of Health
Kingdon, John, 2, 19n1, 134–137,
    142–145, 154, 155, 157, 159
    antecedent policies, 144–145
    New Zealand case study, 134
    and Westminster systems, 71, 136,
        137, 143, 154
    *See also* MS Framework (Multiple
        Streams Framework)
Klein, R., 36
Kusi-Ampofo, O., 16

**L**

Labour, 22–24, 47, 51, 61, 67, 83, 96, 118, 119
Labour government, 49
  in England, 22, 34, 65, 112, 141
  in New Zealand, 25, 81, 97–100, 112, 116, 120, 132, 142
Labour party, 24, 76, 79, 81, 82
  in England, 33, 35, 62
  in New Zealand, 23, 82, 99, 100, 114, 116, 122, 126, 137;
    Manifesto, 12, 24, 76, 79, 81, 82
Landscape, institutional, 72, 104, 113, 121, 122
Laugesen, M., 75
Literature, 2, 5, 27
  on MS Framework, 135–137, 144, 159
  on pay-for-performance, 5, 52, 53, 66, 79
  *See also* Research
Load, 61

**M**

Māori, 76, 78, 79, 88–91, 97, 101, 107, 113, 114, 116–118, 127, 154
McDonald, R., 54
Media, 12, 40, 48, 51, 62, 69, 158
  England, 40, 48, 51, 53, 62, 63, 65
Medical profession, *see* Profession
Method, comparative, 131–134
Minimum Practice Income Guarantee (MPIG), 45
Minister of Health, 27, 82, 95, 98, 126, 130
  *See also* King, Annette
Ministers, 135, 142
  England, 35, 36, 45, 52, 60, 61, 63 (*see also* Hutton)

New Zealand, 93, 98 (*see also* Minister of Health)
Ministry of Health, 25, 28, 77, 82–88, 93, 106
Mintrom, M., ix, 16, 68
Model, 10, 11, 18, 50, 52, 53, 87, 132
  Kingdon, 112, 119 (*see also* MS Framework (Multiple Streams Framework))
  New Zealand, 78, 85, 90, 93, 99, 103, 116, 120, 126
  PRICCE, 42, 53, 61, 67, 101, 131, 147
  Zahariadis, 61, 63, 65–67, 71, 73, 114, 122, 144, 145
MS Framework (Multiple Streams Framework), 134–137, 143–145, 154, 155, 159
Mucciaroni, G., 136

**N**

National Audit Office, 54
National Health Index, 96
National Health Service (NHS), 6n1, 25, 26, 28, 34–36, 51, 60, 61, 101, 126
  Confederation, 47, 65 (*see also* Confederation team)
  contracts, 36, 54
  in media (*see* Media)
  negotiation, 41–43, 47 (*see also* Farrar)
National Health Service Act 1946, 25
National Institute for Health Research, 54
National Institute of Clinical Excellence, 128
National mood, 11, 12, 62, 114
National Party, 79, 116
National Primary Care Research and Development Centre, 41

Needs, 4, 29, 47, 68, 76, 82, 86
  community, local, 28, 29, 54, 83,
    84, 91, 96, 97, 122
  health, 39, 45, 129
  high, 88–91, 94, 105
Negotiations, 61, 62, 64, 67, 68, 129,
    153
  England, 22, 35–39, 41, 47–49, 52,
    62, 63
  principle-based, 42
  See also Bargaining
Networks, 13–15, 73, 126, 140, 141,
    143, 144, 147, 153–155
  See also Zahariadis
New Public Management, 3, 4, 26,
    133, 142
New Zealand Health Strategy, 82–84,
    87
New Zealand Medical Association
    (NZMA), 101
NHS and Community Care Act 1990,
    27
NHS Pay Modernisation, 54
NHS Plan, 34, 44, 46
No. 10, see Blair, Ton

O
OECD, 3, 27
Oliver, T., 16
Otago University Wellington School,
    88, 93
Outcomes, 106, 128–131, 143, 145
  administrative, 128
  health, 26, 87, 120, 126, 128, 131,
    141, 145, 146, 153–155

P
Pacific people, see Māori
Patients, 23–26, 28, 46, 68, 73, 90,
    95, 96, 115, 148

  England, 36, 39, 44, 53, 91; and
    negotiations, 47, 49; and QOF,
    53, 55; and targets, 54
  New Zealand, 76, 83; and PHOs,
    90, 95, 96, 115, 129; needs of,
    29 (see also Needs)
Pay-for-performance, 5, 6, 27, 60, 61,
    84, 88, 96, 103, 115, 136, 142,
    147, 153–155
  and ambiguity, 67, 118
  comparisons, England and NZ, 125,
    132, 133
  England, 34, 35, 40, 63–66, 71, 72,
    141, 147; New Zealand, 84,
    88, 103, 139–141; NZ Health
    Strategy, 84; and primary health
    care, 96; scepticism about, 115
  research, 18, 55, 145, 146
  schemes, 2, 41, 52, 64, 90, 103,
    104, 126, 145–147, 157
  targets, 121, 130
  and theory, 139–141
Performance and Incentive
    Framework, 107, 130
Performance Programme (PP), 92–96,
    102, 106, 107, 128, 130, 131
  entrepreneurs, 116–118
  evaluation and review of, 104–106,
    120
  implementation, 121–122
  and MS Framework, 112
  purpose, 97
Policy, 60, 63–68, 70–73, 117, 122,
    157
  ambiguity, see Ambiguity
  change, 2, 69, 71, 132, 136–139,
    143–145, 155, 157 (see also
    Change, non-incremental)
  design, vi, 38, 95, 119, 121, 122,
    126, 137; process, 72, 73, 117,
    122, 157
  drivers, 125

entrepreneurs, vi, 10–12, 14,
    16–19, 67, 68, 116–118, 135,
    136, 143
  ideas, 11, 13, 14, 60, 63–65, 67,
    70, 114, 115, 144, 146
  network, 14, 15, 19n1, 73
  window, 10, 15–17, 66, 71, 113,
    116, 146, 147
Policymakers, 13, 14, 19, 64, 100,
    107, 131, 141, 144–146, 148
  England, 103, 117
  New Zealand, 4, 73, 88, 140, 142,
    146–148
  pay-for-performance, 2, 44, 60, 61,
    67, 112, 117
  in Westminster systems, 137, 143,
    148
Primary care, 126, 127, 131
  England, 35, 38, 49, 54, 129
  New Zealand, 77, 78, 82–84, 88,
    101, 102, 107
  See also Care, primary health
Primary Care Clinical Effectiveness
    (PRICCE), ), 37, 41, 42, 49, 52,
    53, 61, 67
Primary Care Trust (PCT), 37, 43, 47,
    54
Primary Health Care Strategy (PHCS),
    82–84, 96, 99, 112, 113
Primary Health Organisation (PHO),
    29, 83–87, 91, 92, 94, 95, 128,
    129, 141
  evaluations of, 104–106, 120
  funding, 96, 130
  and IPAs, 93, 98
  performance of, 107
  policy design, 98, 101, 115
Prime Minister (England), see Blair,
    Tony
Profession, 1, 4, 27, 88, 98, 99, 103,
    116, 134, 140, 148

England, 22, 35, 52, 73;
  government/state, 35, 47, 129
New Zealand, 13, 22–25, 81, 103,
  122, 147; and funder, 88, 98;
  and government, 99, 130
and pay-for-performance, 5, 34, 44,
  115
and state, 116, 134, 140


Q
Quality and Outcomes Framework
    (QOF), 36, 38, 42, 46, 50–53,
    145, 146
  achievements, 45, 51, 54–56, 129,
    130
  evaluations and reviews, 54–56
  indicators, 54–56
  negotiation, 47–49, 138
  and PRICCE, 42, 52, 53, 67
  and theory, 70
Quality Management Advisory System
    (QMAS), 43, 64, 72, 106, 129


R
Referred services, 78–80, 86–88, 90,
    107
Referred Services Advisory Group
    (RSAG), 86, 87, 95, 102, 120
Referred Services Expert Advisory
    Group (RSEAG), 88–91
Research, 2, 16, 55, 62, 78, 79, 82,
    131
  on MS Framework, 14, 143 (see also
    Zahariadis)
  on pay-for-performance, 18, 65, 67,
    126
  'this research', 2, 14, 55, 83, 140,
    143, 145–147, 154, 155, 159
  See also Studies

Resources, 11, 14, 18, 67, 107, 113,
 116, 132, 136, 141, 146, 147
Risk, 69, 117, 120, 137

**S**
Salami tactics, 14, 67, 68, 116
Saltman, R., 145
Schemes, 49, 122, 131, 137, 138,
 141, 145
 incentive, 5, 6, 55, 131 (*see also*
 Pay-for-performance)
Schlager, E., 144
Secretary of State for Health, 35, 40,
 126
Snell, T., 37, 48
Soup, primeval, 11, 13, 63, 142
Spohr, F., 17, 143
Starke, P., 142
Stevens, S., 35
Strategies, 12, 14, 27, 67, 68, 76,
 116, 120, 131, 135
 entrepreneur's, 69, 117
 government, 82–83
 negotiating, 34, 43, 68
Streams, 11, 13, 14, 18, 63–65,
 114–116, 146, 155
 policy, 12–15, 63–65, 114–116,
  144; community, 65, 114–116;
  idea, 11, 13, 63–65, 114, 115,
  146
 policy entrepreneurs, 10–12, 16–19,
  67, 68, 112, 113, 116, 118,
  126, 135, 136, 143
 policy window, 10, 12–17, 66, 71,
  113, 118, 146, 147
 politics, 12, 14, 15, 17, 19, 62, 112,
  114, 144
 problems, 12, 61, 70, 113, 114
Studies, 9, 16, 17, 122, 142–144
 comparative, xv, 3, 17, 147
 'this study', vii, 63, 65, 112, 113,
  116, 119, 145

*See also* Case studies
Style, 116, 146, 147
Systems, 3, 17, 19, 34, 35, 44, 46, 66,
 154, 157
 clinical, 85, 87, 89, 92, 115
 governing, 71, 120, 123, 132, 146,
  154
 health, 3, 4, 21, 22, 27, 35, 132,
  145, 158
 payment, 112, 145
 practice management, 64, 102,
  105
 purchasing, 142
 quality, 115, 117
 resourcing and remuneration, 139,
  154
 Westminster, 71, 120, 132,
  135–137, 143, 154, 155
*See also* Data; Information

**T**
Targets, 35, 44, 47, 78, 84, 91, 103,
 128–130
 achieved, 54, 56, 64, 70
 in bargaining, 137, 138
Technology, 18, 60, 112
 information, 54, 105
 unclear, 10, 18, 19, 60, 70, 112,
  116, 118, 134, 135
Theories, 2, 4, 14, 139–142, 144
 MS Framework, 10, 11, 69, 135,
  136
 single, xv, 2, 10, 18, 145
Tuohy, C., 18, 27
 *See also* Entrepreneurs; History,
  England; Westminster systems

**V**
Value acceptability, 12, 13, 15, 63, 64,
 114, 115
Values, 11–13, 42, 64, 80

**W**

Wellington School of Medicine and Health Sciences, 88, 93

Westminster systems, *see* Systems, Westminster

**Z**

Zahariadis, xv, 3, 11, 19, 71, 144
antecedents, historical, 71
factors, structural, 143, 155
model, 63, 70, 71, 73, 114, 122, 144, 145
MS Framework, 14, 15, 44, 155
networks, 11, 13, 15, 139, 140
policy community, 65, 114, 155 (*see also* Zahariadis, networks)
streams, 14, 19, 19n1, 61, 63, 66, 67, 70, 71, 113, 114

Zohlnhöfer, R., 17, 143, 144